OWEN HUNTER

Dermatitis

Your Comprehensive Blueprint for Diagnosis and Treatment

Contents

INTRODUCTION

Dermatitis, a broad term encompassing a group of inflammatory skin conditions, is a prevalent and often frustrating experience for millions of individuals worldwide. From the relentless itch of atopic dermatitis (eczema) to the unsightly rashes of contact dermatitis, these skin disorders can significantly impact a person's quality of life, personal relationships, and overall well-being. As a medical professional with extensive experience in the field of dermatology, I have witnessed firsthand the profound physical and emotional toll that dermatitis can take on patients. It is this deep understanding of the challenges faced by those living with these skin conditions that has motivated me to write this comprehensive guide.

In this book, we will embark on a journey to unravel the complexities of dermatitis, exploring its various forms, underlying causes, and the most effective management strategies. Whether you are a healthcare provider seeking to enhance your clinical knowledge or an individual grappling with the daily struggles of living with dermatitis, this book aims to be your trusted companion, providing you with the tools and insights necessary to navigate this often perplexing skin condition.

Dermatitis: A Widespread and Diverse Skin Disorder

Dermatitis, a term derived from the Greek words "derma" (skin) and "itis" (inflammation), is a broad umbrella term that encompasses a wide range of inflammatory skin conditions. These conditions share a common thread: the skin's immune system becomes overactive, leading to redness, itching, and various other unpleasant symptoms. While the specific causes and manifestations of dermatitis may differ, the underlying theme of skin inflammation unites these diverse skin disorders.

One of the most prevalent forms of dermatitis is atopic dermatitis, also known as eczema. Affecting up to 20% of children and 3% of adults worldwide, atopic dermatitis is characterized by a chronic, relapsing course, marked by intense itching and a characteristic red, scaly rash. The condition is often associated with other atopic disorders, such as asthma and allergic rhinitis, underscoring the complex interplay between the skin and the body's immune system.

Another well-known form of dermatitis is contact dermatitis, which can be further divided into two subtypes: irritant contact dermatitis and allergic contact dermatitis. Irritant contact dermatitis is triggered by direct exposure to irritating substances, such as certain chemicals, soaps, or even water, while allergic contact dermatitis results from an immune system reaction to specific allergens, like nickel or poison ivy. Both forms of contact dermatitis can lead to debilitating skin rashes, blisters, and discomfort.

Seborrheic dermatitis, often characterized by a red, flaky, and sometimes greasy rash, predominantly affects the scalp, face, and other oil-rich areas of the body. This condition is thought to be influenced by a combination of factors, including an overgrowth of a naturally occurring yeast on the skin, hormonal imbalances, and underlying medical conditions.

Dermatitis can also manifest in more specialized forms, such as diaper dermatitis, which affects the delicate skin of infants and toddlers; dermatitis herpetiformis, an autoimmune condition linked to gluten sensitivity; and nummular dermatitis, which presents as distinctive coin-shaped lesions.

The Profound Impact of Dermatitis

The impact of dermatitis extends far beyond the physical symptoms, as these skin conditions can have a significant influence on an individual's emotional, social, and overall quality of life. The relentless itch, unsightly rashes, and discomfort associated with dermatitis can lead to sleep disturbances, anxiety, depression, and social isolation. Individuals with visible skin lesions may face stigma, discrimination, and challenges in professional and personal relationships.

Moreover, the financial burden of dermatitis can be substantial, both for the individual and the healthcare system. Patients may require frequent visits to healthcare providers, extensive treatment regimens, and time off work or school, leading to lost productivity and increased healthcare costs. In the United States alone, the direct and indirect costs associated with atopic dermatitis are estimated to exceed $5 billion annually.

Navigating the Complexities of Dermatitis

Given the diverse nature of dermatitis and the significant impact it can have on an individual's life, it is crucial to approach this condition with a comprehensive understanding. This book is designed to serve as a valuable resource for healthcare professionals, patients, and caregivers, providing in-depth insights into the various forms of dermatitis, their underlying causes, and the most effective management strategies.

Throughout the following chapters, we will delve into the pathophysiology, clinical presentation, and diagnostic criteria of the different types of dermatitis. We will explore the latest advancements in topical and systemic treatments, including traditional pharmacological therapies, as well as emerging options such as biologics and complementary approaches.

Special attention will be given to the management of dermatitis in specific populations, such as infants, children, the elderly, and pregnant individuals, who may require tailored care.

By arming readers with a comprehensive understanding of dermatitis, this book aims to empower individuals to take an active role in their skin health and collaborate with healthcare providers to develop personalized treatment plans. Additionally, we will discuss the importance of preventive measures, lifestyle modifications, and coping strategies to help minimize the burden of these skin conditions and improve overall quality of life.

The Road Ahead

Dermatitis, with its diverse manifestations and complex etiologies, continues to present challenges for healthcare providers and patients alike. However, through ongoing research, evolving treatment modalities, and a deeper understanding of the underlying mechanisms, the management of dermatitis has steadily improved in recent years.

In this book, we will explore the latest advancements in the field of dermatology, highlighting the promising developments that offer hope for more effective and personalized care. By delving into the intricacies of dermatitis, we aim to equip readers with the knowledge and tools necessary to navigate this complex skin condition and ultimately improve the lives of those affected.

Whether you are a healthcare professional seeking to enhance your clinical expertise or an individual living with dermatitis, this book is your comprehensive guide to understanding, managing, and ultimately, overcoming the challenges posed by this diverse and often perplexing skin disorder. Join us on this journey as we unravel the mysteries of dermatitis and empower individuals to take control of their skin health.

CHAPTER 1

U nderstanding Dermatitis

Dermatitis: A Multifaceted Skin Condition

Dermatitis, a term derived from the Greek words "derma" (skin) and "itis" (inflammation), is a broad and complex condition that encompasses a wide range of inflammatory skin disorders. While the specific manifestations and underlying causes may vary, the common thread that unites these diverse skin conditions is the involvement of the skin's immune system, leading to a characteristic pattern of redness, itching, and other unpleasant symptoms.

At its core, dermatitis is a result of the skin's immune system becoming overactive, triggering an inflammatory response that leads to the development of various skin lesions and discomfort. This overreaction of the immune system can be triggered by a multitude of factors, ranging from environmental exposures and genetic predispositions to underlying medical conditions and lifestyle factors.

Deciphering the Types of Dermatitis

Dermatitis is not a singular entity but rather a collective term that encompasses several distinct skin conditions, each with its own unique characteristics, causes, and management approaches. Understanding the different forms of dermatitis is crucial for healthcare providers and patients alike, as it allows for accurate diagnosis, targeted treatment, and effective management of this complex skin disorder.

Atopic Dermatitis (Eczema)

One of the most prevalent forms of dermatitis is atopic dermatitis, commonly known as eczema. Atopic dermatitis is a chronic, relapsing skin condition characterized by intense itching, redness, and a distinctive pattern of skin lesions. This condition is often associated with a personal or family history of other atopic disorders, such as asthma and allergic rhinitis, underscoring the intricate relationship between the skin and the body's immune system.

Atopic dermatitis typically manifests in early childhood, with the majority of cases presenting before the age of 5. However, the condition can persist into adulthood, with flare-ups and remissions occurring throughout an individual's lifetime. Roughly 10-20% of children and 3% of adults worldwide are affected by atopic dermatitis, making it a significant public health concern.

Contact Dermatitis

Another common form of dermatitis is contact dermatitis, which can be further classified into two distinct subtypes: irritant contact dermatitis and allergic contact dermatitis.

Irritant contact dermatitis is caused by direct exposure to irritating substances, such as harsh chemicals, harsh soaps, or even prolonged contact with water. This type of dermatitis is the most prevalent form, accounting for approximately 80% of all contact dermatitis cases. The skin's reaction to these irritants can result in redness, swelling, and a burning or stinging sensation.

Allergic contact dermatitis, on the other hand, is triggered by an immune system reaction to specific allergens, such as nickel, latex, or poison ivy. In this case, the skin develops a delayed hypersensitivity response, leading to a characteristic red, itchy rash that may persist for several days or even weeks after exposure to the allergen.

Seborrheic Dermatitis

Seborrheic dermatitis is another common form of dermatitis, characterized by a red, flaky, and sometimes greasy rash that predominantly affects the scalp, face, and other oil-rich areas of the body. This condition is thought to be influenced by a combination of factors, including an overgrowth of a naturally occurring yeast on the skin, hormonal imbalances, and underlying medical conditions, such as Parkinson's disease or HIV/AIDS.

Seborrheic dermatitis can occur at any age, from infancy to adulthood, and is estimated to affect up to 5% of the general population. While the condition is not contagious, it can be a source of significant discomfort and self-consciousness for those affected.

Other Forms of Dermatitis

In addition to the aforementioned types of dermatitis, there are several other less common but equally important forms of this skin condition, including:

1. Diaper Dermatitis: A form of irritant contact dermatitis that affects the delicate skin of infants and toddlers, often due to prolonged exposure to urine, feces, and skin irritants within the diaper area.

2. Dermatitis Herpetiformis: An autoimmune form of dermatitis characterized by intensely itchy, blistering rashes that are closely associated with celiac disease and gluten sensitivity.

3. Nummular Dermatitis: A distinctive form of dermatitis that presents as coin-shaped lesions, often triggered by dry skin, minor skin injuries, or

underlying conditions.

4. Stasis Dermatitis: A type of dermatitis that occurs due to poor circulation, often seen in individuals with venous insufficiency or other underlying vascular disorders.

5. Perioral Dermatitis: A localized form of dermatitis that affects the skin around the mouth, commonly triggered by the use of topical corticosteroids or other facial products.

Understanding the Causes and Triggers of Dermatitis

The underlying causes and triggers of dermatitis are multifactorial, involving a complex interplay between genetic predispositions, environmental exposures, and various physiological and immunological factors.

Genetic Factors

Certain genetic variations and polymorphisms have been associated with an increased risk of developing specific forms of dermatitis, particularly atopic dermatitis. Studies have identified several genes involved in skin barrier function, immune system regulation, and inflammation that may contribute to the development and progression of atopic dermatitis.

Environmental Exposures

Environmental factors, such as allergens, irritants, and microorganisms, can play a significant role in triggering and exacerbating dermatitis. Allergens, such as dust mites, pollen, or certain foods, can elicit an immune system reaction in individuals with atopic dermatitis, leading to flare-ups. Irritants, including harsh soaps, chemicals, and even water, can disrupt the skin's barrier function and trigger inflammatory responses in various forms of dermatitis.

Microbial imbalances, such as an overgrowth of the Staphylococcus aureus bacteria on the skin, have also been linked to the development and exacerbation of atopic dermatitis. These microbial influences can further contribute to the complex interplay between the skin, immune system, and environmental factors in the pathogenesis of dermatitis.

Immune System Dysregulation

At the core of dermatitis is an overactive and dysregulated immune system. In individuals with dermatitis, the skin's immune cells, such as T cells and mast cells, become hyperresponsive, leading to the release of inflammatory mediators and the development of characteristic skin lesions.

This immune system dysregulation can be influenced by various factors, including genetic predispositions, environmental exposures, and underlying medical conditions. For example, in atopic dermatitis, the skin's immune system becomes hypersensitive to allergens and irritants, triggering a cascade of inflammatory responses.

Skin Barrier Dysfunction

The skin's barrier function, which is responsible for maintaining hydration and protecting the body from external threats, can also play a crucial role in the development of dermatitis. In individuals with dermatitis, the skin's barrier function is often impaired, leading to increased water loss, increased susceptibility to irritants and allergens, and the development of inflammation.

This skin barrier dysfunction can be influenced by genetic factors, environmental exposures, and even the dysregulation of the skin's immune system. For example, in atopic dermatitis, mutations in genes responsible for the production of important skin barrier proteins, such as filaggrin, have been associated with an increased risk of developing the condition.

Underlying Medical Conditions

In some cases, dermatitis may be a manifestation of an underlying medical condition or a complication of certain therapies. For instance, seborrheic dermatitis has been associated with neurological disorders like Parkinson's disease, as well as conditions that affect the immune system, such as HIV/AIDS.

Additionally, certain medications, such as topical corticosteroids, can lead to the development of a form of dermatitis known as perioral dermatitis when used excessively or for prolonged periods.

Recognizing the Symptoms and Diagnostic Criteria

The clinical presentation of dermatitis can vary greatly, depending on the specific type of the condition and the individual's response to various triggers. However, there are some common symptoms and diagnostic criteria that healthcare providers can use to identify and differentiate between the different forms of dermatitis.

Symptoms of Dermatitis
The hallmark symptoms of dermatitis include:

1. Skin redness and inflammation
2. Itching, which can be intense and persistent
3. Scaling, flaking, or dryness of the affected skin
4. Blisters, weeping, or crusting of the skin lesions
5. Thickening or lichenification of the skin in chronic cases

The distribution and pattern of the skin lesions can also provide valuable clues to the specific type of dermatitis. For example, atopic dermatitis typically presents with a characteristic eczematous rash that is often found in the skin creases, such as the elbows, knees, and neck. Contact dermatitis, on the other hand, may exhibit a more localized rash at the site of exposure to the irritant or allergen.

Diagnostic Criteria and Evaluation

Diagnosing dermatitis often involves a comprehensive clinical evaluation, which includes a thorough medical history, physical examination, and, in some cases, additional testing.

Medical History

The healthcare provider will gather information about the patient's symptoms, including the onset, duration, and pattern of the skin lesions, as well as any potential triggers or aggravating factors. They will also inquire about the patient's personal and family history of atopic or other skin conditions, as well as any underlying medical conditions that may be contributing to the dermatitis.

Physical Examination

A detailed physical examination of the skin is crucial for diagnosing dermatitis. The healthcare provider will closely inspect the affected areas, evaluating the characteristics of the skin lesions, such as their appearance, distribution, and severity. They may also perform a skin biopsy in certain cases to rule out other skin conditions or confirm the diagnosis.

Additional Testing

Depending on the suspected type of dermatitis, the healthcare provider may order additional tests to aid in the diagnosis. These may include:

1. Allergy testing (e.g., patch testing, skin prick testing) for suspected cases of contact dermatitis
2. Blood tests to assess for underlying medical conditions or immune system abnormalities
3. Bacterial or fungal cultures to identify any secondary infections
4. Genetic testing for certain forms of dermatitis, such as atopic dermatitis

By combining the patient's medical history, physical examination findings, and any necessary diagnostic tests, healthcare providers can accurately identify the specific type of dermatitis and develop an appropriate treatment plan.

Conclusion

Dermatitis is a complex and multifaceted skin condition that encompasses a wide range of inflammatory disorders, each with its own unique characteristics, causes, and management strategies. Understanding the different types of dermatitis, their underlying mechanisms, and the diagnostic criteria is crucial for healthcare providers and patients alike.

In this chapter, we have explored the various forms of dermatitis, from the prevalent atopic dermatitis to the more specialized conditions like contact dermatitis and seborrheic dermatitis. We have delved into the complex interplay of genetic, environmental, and immunological factors that contribute to the development and progression of these skin disorders.

By gaining a comprehensive understanding of dermatitis, we can lay the foundation for effective management and improved quality of life for those affected by this often perplexing and burdensome skin condition. In the following chapters, we will continue to explore the intricacies of dermatitis, focusing on the specific clinical features, diagnostic approaches, and the latest advancements in treatment options.

CHAPTER 2

Atopic Dermatitis (Eczema)

Atopic dermatitis, often referred to as eczema, is one of the most prevalent and well-known forms of dermatitis. As a chronic, relapsing skin condition, atopic dermatitis is characterized by intense itching, red and inflamed skin, and a distinctive pattern of lesions that can significantly impact an individual's quality of life. Understanding the epidemiology, pathophysiology, and clinical features of atopic dermatitis is crucial for healthcare providers and patients alike, as it lays the foundation for effective diagnosis and management.

Epidemiology and Burden of Atopic Dermatitis

Atopic dermatitis is a global health concern, with a significant and growing prevalence worldwide. It is estimated that up to 20% of children and 3% of adults are affected by this condition, making it one of the most common chronic inflammatory skin disorders.

The incidence of atopic dermatitis appears to be higher in developed countries, with the highest rates reported in the United States, United Kingdom, and Scandinavia. This geographical distribution suggests that environmental and lifestyle factors may play a role in the development and expression of the condition.

The onset of atopic dermatitis typically occurs in early childhood, with the majority of cases presenting before the age of 5. However, the condition can persist into adulthood, with intermittent flare-ups and periods of remission throughout an individual's lifetime. In some cases, the symptoms may improve or even resolve as the child grows older, but a significant proportion of patients continue to experience the condition in adulthood.

The burden of atopic dermatitis extends beyond the physical symptoms, as it can have a profound impact on an individual's emotional, social, and overall quality of life. The relentless itch, unsightly skin lesions, and discomfort associated with the condition can lead to sleep disturbances, anxiety, depression, and social isolation. Individuals with visible skin lesions may face stigma, discrimination, and challenges in professional and personal relationships.

Moreover, the financial burden of atopic dermatitis is substantial, both for the individual and the healthcare system. Patients may require frequent visits to healthcare providers, extensive treatment regimens, and time off work or school, leading to lost productivity and increased healthcare costs. In the United States alone, the direct and indirect costs associated with atopic dermatitis are estimated to exceed $5 billion annually.

Pathophysiology of Atopic Dermatitis

The complex pathophysiology of atopic dermatitis involves a multifaceted interplay between genetic, immunological, and environmental factors. Understanding the underlying mechanisms of this condition is crucial for the development of effective treatment strategies and the identification of potential targets for intervention.

Genetic Factors

Numerous studies have identified genetic variations and polymorphisms that contribute to the development and progression of atopic dermatitis. One of the most well-studied genes associated with the condition is the filaggrin (FLG) gene, which plays a crucial role in the maintenance of the skin's barrier function.

Mutations in the FLG gene can lead to a defective skin barrier, allowing for increased water loss and increased susceptibility to environmental triggers, such as allergens and irritants. This skin barrier dysfunction is believed to be a primary driver in the pathogenesis of atopic dermatitis, as it sets the stage for the development of inflammation and the characteristic skin lesions.

In addition to the FLG gene, other genes involved in immune system regulation, inflammation, and skin barrier function have also been implicated in the genetic predisposition to atopic dermatitis. The interplay between these genetic factors and environmental exposures contributes to the complex and heterogeneous nature of the condition.

Immune System Dysregulation

At the core of atopic dermatitis is an overactive and dysregulated immune system. In individuals with the condition, the skin's immune cells, such as T cells and mast cells, become hyperresponsive, leading to the release of inflammatory mediators and the development of characteristic skin lesions.

The immune system dysregulation in atopic dermatitis is characterized by a predominant T helper type 2 (Th2) immune response, which involves the production of specific cytokines, such as interleukin-4 (IL-4), interleukin-5 (IL-5), and interleukin-13 (IL-13). These Th2 cytokines promote the activation and recruitment of eosinophils, mast cells, and other inflammatory cells, contributing to the inflammation and skin barrier dysfunction observed in atopic dermatitis.

Furthermore, the skin's innate immune system, which acts as the first line of defense against external threats, is also impaired in individuals with atopic dermatitis. This impairment leads to a decreased ability to mount an effective response against microbial pathogens, such as Staphylococcus aureus, which can further exacerbate the skin inflammation and contribute to the development of secondary infections.

Environmental Factors and Triggers

Environmental factors and exposures play a crucial role in the development and exacerbation of atopic dermatitis. Allergens, irritants, and other environmental stimuli can trigger the activation of the skin's immune system, leading to flare-ups and the characteristic skin lesions.

Common environmental triggers for atopic dermatitis include:

1. Allergens: Dust mites, pollen, pet dander, certain foods (e.g., dairy, eggs, soy, wheat)
2. Irritants: Harsh soaps, detergents, chemicals, wool, and synthetic fabrics
3. Stress: Psychological stress can worsen atopic dermatitis by altering the body's immune and hormonal responses
4. Climate and weather: Dry, cold, or hot and humid environments can exacerbate symptoms

The interplay between these environmental factors and the individual's genetic predisposition and immune system dysregulation ultimately contributes to the development and progression of atopic dermatitis.

Clinical Presentation and Diagnostic Criteria

The clinical presentation of atopic dermatitis can vary significantly, depending on the individual's age, severity of the condition, and stage of the disease. However, there are several characteristic features that healthcare providers can use to identify and diagnose this skin condition.

Typical Clinical Features

The hallmark symptoms of atopic dermatitis include:

1. Intense, persistent itching: The itch associated with atopic dermatitis is often described as severe and can significantly disrupt sleep and daily activities.

2. Eczematous skin lesions: The skin lesions in atopic dermatitis typically present as red, inflamed, and scaly patches or plaques. In infants and young children, the lesions often appear on the cheeks, forehead, and extensor surfaces of the extremities. In older children and adults, the lesions tend to affect the flexural areas, such as the elbows, knees, and neck.

3. Chronic or relapsing course: Atopic dermatitis is a chronic, relapsing condition, with periods of flare-ups and remission. The condition can persist throughout an individual's lifetime, although the severity and distribution of the skin lesions may change over time.

4. Age-related distribution: The clinical presentation of atopic dermatitis often varies with the patient's age. In infants and young children, the lesions typically appear on the face, scalp, and extensor surfaces of the extremities. In older children and adults, the lesions tend to affect the flexural areas, such as the elbows, knees, and neck.

5. Dry, sensitive skin: Individuals with atopic dermatitis often have inherently dry, sensitive skin, which can further contribute to the development and exacerbation of the condition.

Diagnostic Criteria

Diagnosing atopic dermatitis typically involves a comprehensive clinical evaluation, including a thorough medical history and physical examination. Healthcare providers may use the following diagnostic criteria to identify and confirm the condition:

1. Presence of pruritic (itchy) skin condition
2. Chronic or relapsing history
3. Typical morphology and distribution of the skin lesions
4. Personal or family history of atopic conditions, such as asthma or allergic rhinitis
5. Onset in early childhood
6. Xerosis (dry skin) and enhanced skin reactivity to environmental triggers

In some cases, healthcare providers may order additional tests, such as allergy testing or skin biopsies, to rule out other skin conditions or identify any underlying triggers or contributing factors.

Stages and Severity of Atopic Dermatitis

Atopic dermatitis can manifest in varying degrees of severity and can progress through different stages throughout an individual's lifetime. Understanding the stages and severity of the condition is crucial for healthcare providers to develop appropriate treatment strategies and monitor the patient's response to therapy.

Stages of Atopic Dermatitis

1. Infantile stage: This stage typically begins in infancy, with the skin lesions often appearing on the cheeks, forehead, and extensor surfaces of the extremities.
2. Childhood stage: As the child grows older, the skin lesions may shift to the flexural areas, such as the elbows, knees, and neck. The condition may also become more chronic and relapsing during this stage.
3. Adolescent and adult stage: In some individuals, the condition may persist or even worsen during adolescence and adulthood, with the skin lesions often affecting the hands, feet, and other areas.

Severity of Atopic Dermatitis

The severity of atopic dermatitis can be assessed based on the extent, intensity, and impact of the skin lesions on the patient's quality of life. Healthcare providers may use various scoring systems, such as the Eczema Area and Severity Index (EASI) or the Scoring Atopic Dermatitis (SCORAD) index, to objectively evaluate the severity of the condition.

1. Mild atopic dermatitis: Characterized by limited involvement of the skin, with occasional flare-ups and minimal impact on the patient's quality of life.
2. Moderate atopic dermatitis: Moderate involvement of the skin, with more frequent flare-ups and a greater impact on the patient's quality of life.
3. Severe atopic dermatitis: Extensive involvement of the skin, with frequent and severe flare-ups, significant impact on the patient's quality of life, and potential for complications.

It is important to note that the severity of atopic dermatitis can fluctuate over time, and individuals may experience periods of exacerbation and remission. Regular monitoring and assessment by healthcare providers are crucial for effective management and tailoring of treatment strategies to the individual's needs.

Comorbidities and Associated Conditions

Individuals with atopic dermatitis often have an increased risk of developing other atopic or inflammatory conditions, known as comorbidities. Understanding the associations between atopic dermatitis and these related conditions is essential for comprehensive patient care and management.

Allergic Conditions

Atopic dermatitis is closely linked to other atopic conditions, such as:

1. Allergic rhinitis (hay fever)
2. Asthma
3. Food allergies
4. Allergic conjunctivitis

The shared genetic and immunological factors that contribute to the development of atopic dermatitis may also predispose individuals to these other allergic conditions. Patients with atopic dermatitis should be routinely screened and monitored for the development of these associated allergies.

Psychological and Psychiatric Conditions

The significant impact of atopic dermatitis on an individual's quality of life can also lead to the development of psychological and psychiatric comorbidities, such as:

1. Anxiety
2. Depression
3. Sleep disturbances
4. Attention-deficit/hyperactivity disorder (ADHD)

The relentless itch, visible skin lesions, and social stigma associated with atopic dermatitis can contribute to the onset or exacerbation of these mental health conditions. Addressing the psychological and emotional aspects of the condition is an integral part of comprehensive atopic dermatitis management.

Other Associated Conditions

In addition to allergic and psychological comorbidities, atopic dermatitis has also been linked to various other health conditions, including:

1. Obesity
2. Metabolic syndrome
3. Cardiovascular diseases
4. Autoimmune disorders

The exact mechanisms underlying these associations are not fully understood, but they may involve shared genetic, immunological, and environmental factors, as well as the impact of chronic inflammation on overall health.

Conclusion

Atopic dermatitis, a chronic and relapsing skin condition, is one of the most prevalent forms of dermatitis, affecting millions of individuals worldwide. Understanding the epidemiology, pathophysiology, and clinical presentation of this condition is crucial for healthcare providers to accurately diagnose and effectively manage this complex skin disorder.

In this chapter, we have delved into the various aspects of atopic dermatitis, from its global burden and impact on quality of life to the underlying genetic, immunological, and environmental factors that contribute to its development and progression. We have also explored the characteristic clinical features and diagnostic criteria that healthcare providers can use to identify and differentiate atopic dermatitis from other skin conditions.

Furthermore, we have discussed the stages and severity of atopic dermatitis, as well as the associated comorbidities and conditions that often accompany this skin condition. This comprehensive understanding lays the foundation for the development of personalized treatment strategies and the implementation of holistic management approaches to address the multifaceted needs of individuals living with atopic dermatitis.

As we continue our journey through the various forms of dermatitis, the insights gained from this chapter on atopic dermatitis will serve as a valuable reference point, enabling healthcare providers and patients to navigate the complexities of this prevalent and often debilitating skin condition.

CHAPTER 3

Contact Dermatitis

Among the diverse forms of dermatitis, contact dermatitis stands out as a unique and prevalent condition, characterized by the skin's inflammatory response to external triggers. This chapter will delve into the intricacies of contact dermatitis, exploring its two main subtypes - irritant contact dermatitis and allergic contact dermatitis - as well as their respective causes, clinical features, and management strategies.

Understanding the Subtypes of Contact Dermatitis

Contact dermatitis is a broad term that encompasses two distinct forms of skin inflammation: irritant contact dermatitis and allergic contact dermatitis. While these subtypes share some common characteristics, their underlying mechanisms, triggers, and clinical presentations differ significantly, requiring tailored approaches for accurate diagnosis and effective management.

Irritant Contact Dermatitis

Irritant contact dermatitis is the more common of the two subtypes, accounting for approximately 80% of all contact dermatitis cases. This form of dermatitis is triggered by direct exposure to irritating substances, leading to a non-immunological inflammatory response in the skin.

The key distinguishing feature of irritant contact dermatitis is the direct, dose-dependent relationship between the exposure to the irritant and the development of the skin lesions. Common irritants that can trigger this condition include:

1. Harsh soaps and detergents
2. Solvents and chemicals
3. Acids and alkalis
4. Prolonged exposure to water or friction
5. Industrial materials, such as cement or metalworking fluids

When the skin is exposed to these irritants, it triggers a cascade of inflammatory responses, leading to the characteristic symptoms of irritant contact dermatitis, such as redness, dryness, and a burning or stinging sensation.

Unlike allergic contact dermatitis, the development of irritant contact dermatitis does not require a prior sensitization or immune system involvement. Instead, the severity of the skin reaction is directly proportional to the concentration and duration of exposure to the irritant.

Allergic Contact Dermatitis

Allergic contact dermatitis, on the other hand, is the result of an acquired, cell-mediated immune reaction to specific allergens. In this subtype, the skin's immune system becomes hypersensitive to certain substances, triggering an inflammatory response upon subsequent exposure.

The development of allergic contact dermatitis involves a two-stage process:

1. Sensitization: During the initial exposure to the allergen, the skin's immune system, specifically the T cells, becomes sensitized and recognizes the substance as a foreign invader.

2. Elicitation: Upon subsequent exposure to the same allergen, the sensitized immune system mounts a rapid and exaggerated inflammatory response, leading to the characteristic skin lesions of allergic contact dermatitis.

Common allergens that can trigger this condition include:

1. Metals (e.g., nickel, chromium, cobalt)
2. Fragrances and preservatives
3. Latex
4. Poison ivy and other plants
5. Certain medications applied to the skin

Unlike irritant contact dermatitis, the skin reaction in allergic contact dermatitis is delayed, typically appearing several hours to days after exposure to the allergen. This delayed response is a hallmark feature that distinguishes it from the more immediate reaction seen in irritant contact dermatitis.

Epidemiology and Risk Factors

Contact dermatitis, as a whole, is one of the most common skin conditions, affecting up to 20% of the general population at some point in their lives. The specific prevalence and incidence of the two subtypes, however, can vary based on various factors.

Irritant Contact Dermatitis

Irritant contact dermatitis is the more prevalent form, with an estimated lifetime incidence of up to 70% in the general population. Certain occupations and industries, such as healthcare, construction, and manufacturing, have a higher risk of exposure to irritants, resulting in a higher prevalence of irritant contact dermatitis among these workers.

Additionally, individuals with inherently dry or sensitive skin, as well as those with a history of atopic dermatitis, may be more susceptible to developing irritant contact dermatitis due to their compromised skin barrier function.

Allergic Contact Dermatitis

Allergic contact dermatitis, while less common than its irritant counterpart, still affects a significant portion of the population. The lifetime prevalence of allergic contact dermatitis is estimated to be around 15-20% in the general population, with some variations across different regions and demographics.

Certain occupations, such as healthcare workers, hairdressers, and metal-workers, have a higher risk of exposure to potential allergens, leading to an increased incidence of allergic contact dermatitis in these professions. Additionally, individuals with a personal or family history of atopic dermatitis or other allergic conditions may have a greater predisposition to developing allergic contact dermatitis.

Clinical Presentation and Diagnosis

The clinical presentation of contact dermatitis can vary significantly, depending on the specific subtype, the nature of the exposure, and the individual's response to the triggering agent. However, there are some characteristic features that healthcare providers can use to differentiate between irritant and allergic contact dermatitis.

Irritant Contact Dermatitis

The skin lesions in irritant contact dermatitis are typically well-defined, localized, and directly correspond to the area of exposure to the irritant. The affected skin may appear red, dry, and scaly, with a burning or stinging sensation. In severe cases, the skin may develop blisters, crusting, or even fissures.

The onset of symptoms in irritant contact dermatitis is usually rapid, often occurring within minutes to hours of exposure to the irritant. The severity of the skin reaction is directly proportional to the concentration and duration of exposure, with more intense or prolonged exposure leading to more severe lesions.

Allergic Contact Dermatitis

In contrast, the skin lesions in allergic contact dermatitis may have a more diffuse and widespread distribution, not necessarily limited to the exact area of exposure. The affected skin often appears red, swollen, and itchy, with the development of characteristic eczematous patches or plaques.

The onset of symptoms in allergic contact dermatitis is typically delayed, with the skin reaction appearing several hours to days after exposure to the allergen. This delayed response is a distinguishing feature that helps differentiate allergic contact dermatitis from the more immediate reaction seen in irritant contact dermatitis.

Diagnostic Evaluation

Diagnosing contact dermatitis often involves a combination of a thorough medical history, physical examination, and specialized testing, such as patch testing.

Medical History

The healthcare provider will collect detailed information about the patient's symptoms, including the onset, duration, and pattern of the skin lesions. They will also inquire about any potential exposures to irritants or allergens, both in the workplace and in the patient's daily life.

Physical Examination

A careful physical examination of the skin is essential for identifying the characteristic features of contact dermatitis. The healthcare provider will evaluate the distribution, morphology, and severity of the skin lesions, as well as any associated symptoms, such as itching or pain.

Patch Testing

In cases where the specific trigger for the contact dermatitis is not readily apparent, the healthcare provider may perform a patch test. This diagnostic procedure involves applying small amounts of various potential allergens to the patient's skin and monitoring the skin's reaction over several days.

The results of the patch test can help identify the specific allergen(s) responsible for the patient's allergic contact dermatitis, guiding the development of an effective avoidance and management strategy.

Occupational and Environmental Considerations

Given the nature of contact dermatitis, it is crucial to consider the patient's occupational and environmental exposures when evaluating and managing this condition. The identification and mitigation of these triggers are essential for the successful treatment and prevention of contact dermatitis.

Occupational Exposure

Certain occupations, such as healthcare, construction, and manufacturing, carry a higher risk of exposure to irritants and allergens that can trigger contact dermatitis. Healthcare workers, for example, may be exposed to a variety of chemicals, cleaning agents, and latex, putting them at an increased risk of developing both irritant and allergic contact dermatitis.

When evaluating a patient with contact dermatitis, the healthcare provider should carefully assess the patient's occupation and work environment, including the specific materials, chemicals, and tasks involved. This information can help pinpoint the potential trigger(s) and guide the development of appropriate preventive measures and treatment strategies.

Environmental Exposure

In addition to occupational exposures, individuals may also encounter irritants and allergens in their daily lives that can contribute to the development of contact dermatitis. Common environmental triggers include:

1. Household cleaners and personal care products
2. Jewelry and accessories containing metals
3. Certain plants, such as poison ivy or poison oak
4. Seasonal changes and exposure to outdoor allergens

By gathering a detailed history of the patient's daily activities, living environment, and potential exposures, the healthcare provider can better identify the underlying cause(s) of the contact dermatitis and develop a comprehensive management plan.

Management and Treatment Strategies

The management of contact dermatitis typically involves a multifaceted approach, focusing on the identification and avoidance of the triggering agent, as well as the use of appropriate topical and systemic therapies to alleviate the symptoms and promote skin healing.

Identification and Avoidance of Triggers

The primary goal in the management of contact dermatitis is to identify and eliminate the underlying trigger, whether it be an irritant or an allergen. This can involve:

1. Thorough history-taking and physical examination to pinpoint the suspected trigger
2. Patch testing or other diagnostic procedures to confirm the specific allergen(s)

3. Providing education and guidance to the patient on how to avoid or minimize exposure to the identified trigger(s)

In the case of occupational contact dermatitis, this may require changes in the work environment, the use of protective equipment, or even job reassignment to minimize exposure to the offending agent.

Topical Treatments

Once the trigger has been identified and exposure has been minimized, the healthcare provider can focus on the use of topical therapies to manage the skin lesions and alleviate the symptoms of contact dermatitis.

1. Emollients and moisturizers: These help restore the skin's barrier function and prevent further irritation.
2. Topical corticosteroids: These anti-inflammatory agents can effectively reduce the redness, itching, and swelling associated with contact dermatitis.
3. Calcineurin inhibitors: These immunomodulatory agents, such as tacrolimus and pimecrolimus, can be used as an alternative to corticosteroids in certain cases.

The healthcare provider will tailor the topical treatment regimen to the specific needs of the patient, taking into account the severity of the condition, the location of the skin lesions, and the patient's response to the therapy.

Systemic Treatments

In more severe or widespread cases of contact dermatitis, the healthcare provider may consider the use of systemic therapies, such as:

1. Oral antihistamines: These can help alleviate the itching and other symptoms associated with the skin condition.
2. Oral corticosteroids: In cases of severe or debilitating contact dermatitis, short-term use of oral corticosteroids may be warranted to quickly control the inflammation.
3. Immunosuppressants: In refractory or chronic cases, the healthcare provider may prescribe oral or injectable immunosuppressant medications, such as methotrexate or dupilumab, to modulate the underlying immune response.

The decision to use systemic treatments is based on the individual patient's response to topical therapies, the extent and severity of the skin lesions, and the impact of the condition on the patient's quality of life.

Prevention and Lifestyle Modifications

In addition to the treatment of active contact dermatitis, healthcare providers should also emphasize the importance of preventive measures and lifestyle modifications to minimize the risk of future flare-ups.

1. Skin care and bathing routines: Gentle cleansers, lukewarm water, and the use of moisturizers can help maintain the skin's barrier function and prevent irritation.
2. Avoidance of known triggers: Patients should be educated on how to identify and avoid exposure to the specific irritants or allergens that trigger their contact dermatitis.
3. Protective equipment and clothing: The use of protective gloves, aprons, or other clothing can help shield the skin from exposure to potential triggers in the workplace or during daily activities.
4. Stress management: Reducing stress and anxiety, which can exacerbate contact dermatitis, through techniques like meditation, yoga, or counseling may be beneficial.

By incorporating these preventive strategies and lifestyle modifications, patients with contact dermatitis can better manage their condition, reduce the risk of flare-ups, and improve their overall quality of life.

Conclusion

Contact dermatitis, with its two distinct subtypes of irritant and allergic contact dermatitis, is a complex and prevalent skin condition that requires a comprehensive understanding for effective management. In this chapter, we have explored the unique characteristics, epidemiology, and clinical presentation of these two forms of contact dermatitis, as well as the diagnostic approaches healthcare providers can utilize to differentiate between them.

Recognizing the importance of occupational and environmental exposures in the development of contact dermatitis, we have discussed the crucial role of identifying and avoiding the underlying triggers, whether they are irritants or allergens. Additionally, we have outlined the various topical and systemic treatment options, as well as the significance of preventive measures and lifestyle modifications, in the holistic management of this skin condition.

By equipping healthcare providers and patients with a deeper understanding of contact dermatitis, this chapter aims to empower individuals to take an active role in the prevention, diagnosis, and management of this often challenging and disruptive skin condition. As we continue our journey through the diverse forms of dermatitis, the insights gained here will serve as a valuable foundation for the comprehensive care and support of those affected by this prevalent skin disorder.

CHAPTER 4

Seborrheic Dermatitis

Seborrheic dermatitis is a common inflammatory skin condition that primarily affects the scalp, face, and other oil-rich areas of the body. This chronic and relapsing disorder is characterized by a red, flaky, and often greasy rash that can cause significant discomfort and self-consciousness for those affected. In this chapter, we will delve into the underlying causes and predisposing factors of seborrheic dermatitis, explore its clinical features and diagnostic criteria, and discuss the various management strategies aimed at providing relief and improving the overall quality of life for patients.

Understanding the Causes and Predisposing Factors

The exact etiology of seborrheic dermatitis is not fully understood, but it is believed to be influenced by a complex interplay of several factors, including the following:

Yeast Overgrowth

One of the primary factors contributing to the development of seborrheic dermatitis is an overgrowth of a naturally occurring yeast, Malassezia (formerly known as Pityrosporum), on the skin. This lipophilic yeast is found in the sebum-rich areas of the body and is thought to play a crucial role in the pathogenesis of seborrheic dermatitis.

The overgrowth of Malassezia is believed to trigger an inflammatory response in the skin, leading to the characteristic red, flaky, and greasy lesions. This association is further supported by the fact that antifungal treatments targeting Malassezia can be effective in the management of seborrheic dermatitis.

Hormonal Factors

Hormonal imbalances and fluctuations may also contribute to the development and exacerbation of seborrheic dermatitis. The condition is often more prevalent and severe during periods of hormonal changes, such as puberty, pregnancy, and menopause, suggesting a potential link between hormonal factors and the expression of the disease.

The sebaceous glands, which are responsible for producing sebum, are known to be influenced by hormones. An increase in sebum production, as seen during hormonal changes, may create a favorable environment for the overgrowth of Malassezia, ultimately leading to the development of seborrheic dermatitis.

Neurological Conditions

Certain neurological disorders, such as Parkinson's disease, have been associated with an increased risk of developing seborrheic dermatitis. The exact mechanism underlying this association is not entirely clear, but it is thought to involve the disruption of the autonomic nervous system, which can influence the function of the sebaceous glands and the skin's immune responses.

Additionally, conditions that affect the central nervous system, such as stroke, traumatic brain injury, and HIV/AIDS, have also been linked to an increased incidence of seborrheic dermatitis. The precise role of the nervous system in the pathogenesis of this skin condition is an area of ongoing research.

Genetic and Environmental Factors

While the genetic predisposition to seborrheic dermatitis is not as well-established as in other forms of dermatitis, such as atopic dermatitis, there is some evidence that genetic factors may play a role in the development of the condition.

Environmental factors, such as climate and season, may also influence the onset and severity of seborrheic dermatitis. The condition is often reported to be more prevalent in warm and humid climates, as well as during periods of increased stress or change in the environment.

It is important to note that the underlying causes of seborrheic dermatitis are multifactorial, and the interplay between these various factors, including the overgrowth of Malassezia, hormonal influences, neurological conditions, and genetic and environmental elements, contributes to the complex nature of this skin disorder.

Clinical Presentation and Diagnostic Criteria

Seborrheic dermatitis manifests with a characteristic set of clinical features that can help healthcare providers differentiate it from other skin conditions. Understanding the typical presentation and distribution of the lesions is crucial for accurate diagnosis and appropriate management.

Clinical Characteristics
The hallmark features of seborrheic dermatitis include:

1. Erythema (redness): The affected areas of the skin typically appear red or inflamed.
2. Scaling and flakiness: The skin lesions are characterized by the presence of yellowish or whitish, greasy-looking scales or flakes.
3. Oiliness and greasiness: The affected areas often appear shiny, oily, or greasy due to the increased sebum production.

4. Itching: Patients with seborrheic dermatitis may experience mild to moderate itching, although the intensity can vary.

The distribution of the skin lesions is typically concentrated in the sebum-rich areas of the body, including:

1. Scalp: Seborrheic dermatitis is often most prominent on the scalp, where it can present as dandruff or a more severe, scaly rash.
2. Face: The lesions commonly appear on the central face, including the eyebrows, nose, and around the mouth.
3. Ears: The skin within and around the external ear canal may be affected.
4. Chest and upper back: These areas, which have a high concentration of sebaceous glands, can also develop seborrheic dermatitis.
5. Flexural areas: In some cases, the skin folds, such as the armpits and groin, may be involved.

Diagnostic Criteria

Diagnosing seborrheic dermatitis typically involves a comprehensive clinical evaluation, including a thorough medical history and physical examination. Healthcare providers may use the following diagnostic criteria to identify and confirm the condition:

1. Presence of erythema and scaling in the characteristic sebum-rich areas of the body
2. Greasy or oily appearance of the affected skin
3. Pruritus (itching) associated with the skin lesions
4. Chronic or relapsing nature of the condition
5. Exclusion of other skin conditions that may present with similar features

In some cases, healthcare providers may perform additional tests, such as skin biopsies or fungal cultures, to rule out other underlying conditions or to confirm the presence of Malassezia on the skin.

Stages and Severity of Seborrheic Dermatitis

Seborrheic dermatitis can present with varying degrees of severity and may progress through different stages over the course of the individual's lifetime. Understanding the stages and severity of the condition is crucial for healthcare providers to develop appropriate treatment strategies and monitor the patient's response to therapy.

Stages of Seborrheic Dermatitis

1. Infantile stage: Seborrheic dermatitis can manifest in infancy, often presenting as a cradle cap, characterized by a thick, yellow, greasy scale on the scalp.
2. Childhood stage: The condition may persist or reappear during childhood, with the skin lesions typically affecting the scalp, face, and other sebum-rich areas.
3. Adolescent and adult stage: Seborrheic dermatitis can continue into adulthood, with the skin lesions often appearing on the scalp, face, and other areas of the body.

Severity of Seborrheic Dermatitis

The severity of seborrheic dermatitis can be assessed based on the extent, intensity, and impact of the skin lesions on the patient's quality of life. Healthcare providers may use various assessment tools, such as the Seborrheic Dermatitis Area and Severity Index (SDASI), to objectively evaluate the severity of the condition.

1. Mild seborrheic dermatitis: Characterized by limited involvement of the skin, with occasional flare-ups and minimal impact on the patient's quality of life.
2. Moderate seborrheic dermatitis: Moderate involvement of the skin, with more frequent flare-ups and a greater impact on the patient's quality of life.
3. Severe seborrheic dermatitis: Extensive involvement of the skin, with frequent and severe flare-ups, significant impact on the patient's quality of life, and potential for complications.

It is important to note that the severity of seborrheic dermatitis can fluctuate over time, and individuals may experience periods of exacerbation and remission. Regular monitoring and assessment by healthcare providers are crucial for effective management and tailoring of treatment strategies to the individual's needs.

Comorbidities and Associated Conditions

Seborrheic dermatitis is not an isolated skin condition, as it has been associated with various other medical conditions and disorders. Understanding these comorbidities and associated conditions is essential for comprehensive patient care and management.

Neurological Conditions

One of the most well-established associations with seborrheic dermatitis is the presence of certain neurological conditions, particularly Parkinson's disease. The exact mechanisms linking these conditions are not fully understood, but it is believed that the disruption of the autonomic nervous system and the associated hormonal changes may contribute to the development of seborrheic dermatitis.

Other neurological disorders, such as stroke, traumatic brain injury, and

HIV/AIDS, have also been linked to an increased risk of developing seborrheic dermatitis. The impact of these conditions on the skin's function and the nervous system's regulation of sebum production may play a role in the pathogenesis of the skin disorder.

Immunological Conditions

Individuals with compromised or dysregulated immune systems, such as those with HIV/AIDS or organ transplant recipients taking immunosuppressant medications, are at a higher risk of developing seborrheic dermatitis. The underlying immune system dysfunction may contribute to the overgrowth of Malassezia and the subsequent development of the skin condition.

Additionally, conditions that are associated with overall immune system impairment, such as diabetes and certain types of cancer, have been observed to have a higher prevalence of seborrheic dermatitis among affected individuals.

Other Associated Conditions

In addition to the neurological and immunological conditions, seborrheic dermatitis has also been linked to other medical disorders, including:

1. Acne vulgaris: There is a potential association between seborrheic dermatitis and the development of acne, likely due to the shared involvement of the sebaceous glands.
2. Rosacea: Some studies have suggested a potential link between seborrheic dermatitis and the development of rosacea, another common inflammatory skin condition.
3. Psoriasis: In rare cases, seborrheic dermatitis and psoriasis may coexist, leading to a condition known as sebopsoriasis, which can complicate the management of both conditions.

Recognizing and addressing these comorbidities and associated conditions is crucial for healthcare providers to develop a comprehensive treatment plan and ensure optimal management of the patient's overall health.

Management and Treatment Strategies

The management of seborrheic dermatitis typically involves a multifaceted approach, focusing on the use of topical therapies, the management of underlying conditions, and lifestyle modifications to control the symptoms and prevent recurrence.

Topical Treatments

The primary treatment for seborrheic dermatitis involves the use of topical agents that target the underlying causes of the condition, such as the overgrowth of Malassezia and the associated inflammation.

1. Antifungal agents: Topical antifungal medications, such as ketoconazole, selenium sulfide, or zinc pyrithione, can help control the Malassezia overgrowth and reduce the severity of the skin lesions.
2. Corticosteroids: Topical corticosteroids, ranging from mild to potent formulations, can be used to reduce the inflammation and itching associated with seborrheic dermatitis.
3. Calcineurin inhibitors: These immunomodulatory agents, such as tacrolimus or pimecrolimus, may be used as an alternative to corticosteroids in certain cases, particularly on the face or other sensitive areas.
4. Keratolytic agents: Topical agents containing ingredients like salicylic acid or coal tar can help promote the shedding of the scaly, flaky skin associated with seborrheic dermatitis.

The healthcare provider will tailor the topical treatment regimen to the individual patient's needs, considering the severity of the condition, the location of the skin lesions, and the patient's response to the therapy.

Systemic Treatments

In some cases, particularly in severe or refractory cases of seborrheic dermatitis, the healthcare provider may consider the use of systemic therapies in addition to topical treatments.

1. Oral antifungal medications: Oral antifungal drugs, such as itraconazole or fluconazole, may be prescribed to target the Malassezia overgrowth more effectively in widespread or resistant cases.
2. Immunosuppressants: In patients with severe or chronic seborrheic dermatitis, the healthcare provider may prescribe oral or injectable immunosuppressant medications, such as methotrexate or dupilumab, to modulate the underlying immune response and reduce inflammation.

The decision to use systemic treatments is based on the individual patient's response to topical therapies, the extent and severity of the skin lesions, and the impact of the condition on the patient's quality of life.

Management of Underlying Conditions

In cases where seborrheic dermatitis is associated with an underlying medical condition, such as Parkinson's disease or HIV/AIDS, the healthcare provider will also focus on the management of the underlying disorder.

1. Neurological conditions: Proper management of the underlying neurological condition, in collaboration with a neurologist, may help improve the symptoms of seborrheic dermatitis.
2. Immunological conditions: Addressing the underlying immune system dysfunction, through appropriate treatments or management of the

associated condition, can help mitigate the development and severity of seborrheic dermatitis.

By addressing the underlying medical conditions, healthcare providers can not only improve the management of seborrheic dermatitis but also enhance the overall well-being of the patient.

Lifestyle Modifications and Supportive Care

In addition to the medical treatments, healthcare providers should also emphasize the importance of lifestyle modifications and supportive care to help manage seborrheic dermatitis and prevent recurrence.

1. Gentle skin care: Recommending the use of mild, non-irritating cleansers and moisturizers can help maintain the skin's barrier function and prevent further irritation.
2. Sun protection: Encouraging the use of sunscreen, particularly in areas affected by seborrheic dermatitis, can help reduce the risk of flare-ups.
3. Stress management: Incorporating stress-reducing techniques, such as meditation, yoga, or counseling, may help mitigate the impact of stress on the condition.
4. Dietary modifications: While the role of diet in the management of seborrheic dermatitis is not well-established, some patients may benefit from adjusting their intake of certain foods or supplements.

By incorporating these lifestyle modifications and supportive care strategies, patients with seborrheic dermatitis can better manage their condition, reduce the risk of flare-ups, and improve their overall quality of life.

Conclusion

Seborrheic dermatitis is a common and often chronic skin condition that primarily affects the sebum-rich areas of the body, including the scalp, face, and upper trunk. In this chapter, we have explored the complex and multifactorial nature of the condition, delving into the underlying causes and predisposing factors, such as the overgrowth of Malassezia, hormonal influences, and neurological conditions.

We have also discussed the characteristic clinical presentation of seborrheic dermatitis, including the typical distribution and severity of the skin lesions, as well as the diagnostic criteria that healthcare providers can utilize to differentiate this condition from other skin disorders.

Furthermore, we have highlighted the importance of recognizing the comorbidities and associated conditions that may accompany seborrheic dermatitis, as this knowledge is crucial for providing comprehensive patient care and addressing the various aspects of the individual's health.

Finally, we have outlined the multifaceted management strategies for seborrheic dermatitis, focusing on the use of topical and systemic therapies, the management of underlying medical conditions, and the implementation of lifestyle modifications and supportive care. By adopting a holistic approach to the treatment and prevention of seborrheic dermatitis, healthcare providers can help patients achieve better control over their condition and improve their overall quality of life.

As we continue our exploration of the diverse forms of dermatitis, the insights gained in this chapter on seborrheic dermatitis will serve as a valuable foundation for healthcare providers and patients alike, empowering them to navigate the complexities of this prevalent and often persistent skin disorder.

CHAPTER 5

Diaper Dermatitis

Diaper dermatitis, also known as diaper rash or nappy rash, is a common form of irritant contact dermatitis that primarily affects infants and toddlers. This skin condition can cause significant discomfort and distress for both the child and the caregivers. In this chapter, we will delve into the etiology and risk factors associated with diaper dermatitis, explore the clinical presentation and diagnostic considerations, and discuss the various prevention and management strategies that healthcare providers and caregivers can employ to alleviate and mitigate this troublesome skin condition.

Understanding the Etiology of Diaper Dermatitis

Diaper dermatitis is a type of irritant contact dermatitis, which arises from the direct exposure of the delicate skin within the diaper area to various irritants. The primary factors contributing to the development of diaper dermatitis include:

Prolonged Exposure to Urine and Feces

The skin in the diaper area is in constant contact with urine and feces, which can contain a variety of irritants, such as enzymes, acids, and bacteria. This prolonged exposure can disrupt the skin's natural barrier function, leading to inflammation and the development of a rash.

Occlusion and Moisture

The diaper itself, when worn for extended periods, creates a warm, moist, and occluded environment that can further exacerbate the skin's exposure to irritants and promote the growth of microorganisms, such as Candida species.

Friction and Mechanical Irritation

The repeated friction and rubbing of the diaper against the delicate skin in the diaper area can also contribute to the development of diaper dermatitis, causing mechanical irritation and inflammation.

Chemical Irritants

Some ingredients in diaper products, such as fragrances, preservatives, or detergent residues, can act as chemical irritants and trigger an inflammatory response in the skin.

Microorganisms

The warm, moist environment created by the diaper can also promote the growth of microorganisms, such as Candida species, which can further contribute to the development and exacerbation of diaper dermatitis.

Risk Factors and Predisposing Conditions

While diaper dermatitis is a common occurrence in infants and toddlers, certain factors can increase the risk of developing this skin condition or contribute to its severity. Understanding these risk factors is crucial for healthcare providers and caregivers to implement preventive measures and provide appropriate management strategies.

Age

Diaper dermatitis is most prevalent in infants and toddlers, with the highest incidence occurring in the first year of life. This is likely due to the increased susceptibility of the delicate skin in this age group, as well as the more frequent diaper changes and exposure to irritants.

Diarrhea or Loose Stools

Infants and toddlers experiencing diarrhea or loose stools are at a higher risk of developing diaper dermatitis, as the increased moisture and exposure to digestive enzymes can further irritate the skin.

Antibiotic Use

The use of antibiotics, either in the infant or the breastfeeding mother, can disrupt the natural balance of the skin's microbiome, leading to an overgrowth of Candida species and an increased risk of fungal diaper dermatitis.

Atopic Dermatitis

Infants and children with a history of atopic dermatitis (eczema) may be more prone to developing diaper dermatitis due to their inherently sensitive and compromised skin barrier function.

Improper Diapering Techniques

Caregivers who do not follow proper diapering and skin care practices, such as failing to change diapers promptly or using harsh cleansers, may inadvertently contribute to the development or worsening of diaper dermatitis.

Clinical Presentation and Diagnostic Considerations

Diaper dermatitis typically presents with a characteristic set of skin lesions and symptoms that can help healthcare providers and caregivers recognize and distinguish this condition from other skin disorders.

Clinical Characteristics

The hallmark features of diaper dermatitis include:

1. Erythema (redness): The skin in the diaper area appears red and inflamed, often with a well-defined border.
2. Papules and pustules: Small, raised bumps or blisters may develop, especially in cases of fungal or bacterial superinfection.
3. Scaling and peeling: The affected skin may exhibit flaky, peeling, or cracked areas.
4. Burning and irritation: Infants and toddlers with diaper dermatitis may exhibit discomfort, fussiness, and reluctance to have their diapers changed.

The distribution of the skin lesions is typically confined to the areas covered by the diaper, such as the buttocks, genitalia, and inner thighs. In severe or prolonged cases, the rash may extend beyond the diaper area.

Diagnostic Considerations

Diagnosing diaper dermatitis typically involves a thorough clinical evaluation and assessment of the patient's history. Healthcare providers may consider the following diagnostic criteria:

1. Presence of erythema, papules, and/or scaling in the diaper area
2. Temporal association with the use of diapers or incontinence
3. Exclusion of other skin conditions that may present with similar features, such as psoriasis or seborrheic dermatitis

In some cases, the healthcare provider may perform additional tests, such as fungal cultures or skin biopsies, to rule out the presence of secondary infections or underlying conditions.

It is important to note that while diaper dermatitis is a common and often straightforward diagnosis, healthcare providers should be mindful of the potential for more severe or atypical presentations, which may require further investigation and management.

Prevention and Management Strategies

The prevention and management of diaper dermatitis involve a multifaceted approach that focuses on maintaining skin health, minimizing exposure to irritants, and addressing any underlying factors that may contribute to the development or exacerbation of the condition.

Prevention Strategies

Effective prevention of diaper dermatitis involves the implementation of proper diapering and skin care practices, as well as the consideration of certain lifestyle and environmental factors.

1. Frequent diaper changes: Changing diapers promptly, as soon as they become wet or soiled, can help reduce the skin's exposure to urine, feces, and other irritants.
2. Gentle cleansing: Using mild, fragrance-free cleansers and avoiding harsh scrubbing or wiping can help maintain the skin's barrier function.
3. Proper drying: Gently patting the skin dry after cleaning, rather than rubbing, can help prevent further irritation.
4. Barrier ointments: Applying a thin layer of a barrier ointment, such as zinc oxide or petroleum jelly, can create a protective layer on the skin and prevent irritants from further damaging the skin.
5. Breathable fabrics: Choosing diapers and clothing made of natural, breathable materials can help reduce the risk of occlusion and moisture buildup.
6. Avoiding irritants: Identifying and minimizing exposure to potential irritants, such as fragrances, preservatives, or detergent residues, can help prevent the development of diaper dermatitis.

Management Strategies

In the event of diaper dermatitis, a comprehensive management approach should be implemented to address the underlying causes and promote skin healing.

1. Topical treatments:

- Barrier ointments: Zinc oxide, petroleum jelly, or dimethicone-based products can help protect the skin and create a barrier against irritants.

- Antifungal creams: In cases of suspected fungal infections, such as Candida, antifungal creams containing ingredients like nystatin or miconazole may be prescribed.

- Topical corticosteroids: Mild, low-potency topical corticosteroids may be used temporarily to reduce inflammation and accelerate healing, but their use should be monitored closely.

2. Oral treatments:

- Antifungal medications: In severe or recurrent cases of fungal diaper dermatitis, the healthcare provider may prescribe oral antifungal drugs, such as fluconazole or itraconazole.

3. Lifestyle modifications:

- Frequent diaper changes: Ensuring that diapers are changed promptly and the skin is cleaned gently can help prevent further irritation.

- Skin-soothing baths: Allowing the infant or toddler to soak in a warm, oatmeal-based bath can help alleviate discomfort and promote healing.

- Exposure to air: Providing "diaper-free" time, when the child is not wearing a diaper, can help the skin dry out and reduce the risk of occlusion.

4. Addressing underlying conditions:

- Managing diarrhea or loose stools: Treating the underlying cause of diarrhea, such as infection or dietary changes, can help prevent further irritation.

- Monitoring antibiotic use: Carefully monitoring the use of antibiotics and considering probiotic or antifungal supplementation may help maintain a healthy skin microbiome.

- Addressing atopic dermatitis: Treating any co-existing atopic dermatitis can help strengthen the skin's barrier function and reduce the risk of diaper dermatitis.

Caregiver Education and Support

Educating caregivers on the prevention and management of diaper dermatitis is crucial for ensuring the effective and consistent implementation of the necessary strategies. Healthcare providers should:

1. Provide clear instructions on proper diapering and skin care techniques.
2. Offer guidance on the selection and use of appropriate diaper products and skin care products.
3. Emphasize the importance of prompt diaper changes and the need to address any underlying conditions that may contribute to the development of diaper dermatitis.
4. Offer support and resources for caregivers to help them manage the emotional and practical aspects of dealing with this skin condition in their children.

By empowering caregivers with the knowledge and tools to prevent and manage diaper dermatitis, healthcare providers can help alleviate the burden on both the child and the family, ultimately improving the overall well-being and quality of life.

Complications and Considerations

While diaper dermatitis is a common and often manageable skin condition, it can lead to more severe complications or may require special considerations in certain cases.

Secondary Infections

The compromised skin barrier and the warm, moist environment created by the diaper can provide an opportunistic environment for the development of secondary infections, such as:

1. Candidiasis: An overgrowth of Candida species, which can lead to the formation of papules, pustules, and a characteristic "satellite" rash.
2. Bacterial infections: Bacterial pathogens, such as Staphylococcus or Streptococcus, can cause further inflammation and the development of weeping, crusted lesions.

In such cases, the healthcare provider may need to prescribe antifungal or antibiotic medications, in addition to the standard management strategies, to address the secondary infection.

Severe or Recalcitrant Diaper Dermatitis

In some instances, diaper dermatitis may be severe, extensive, or resistant to standard treatment approaches. This may occur in cases of:

1. Underlying skin conditions: Infants or toddlers with pre-existing conditions, such as atopic dermatitis or ichthyosis, may experience more severe and persistent diaper dermatitis.
2. Immunocompromised states: Children with impaired immune function, due to conditions like HIV/AIDS or cancer treatments, may be more susceptible to severe and recalcitrant diaper dermatitis.
3. Genetic or metabolic disorders: Certain genetic or metabolic disorders can predispose individuals to the development of intractable diaper dermatitis.

In these complex cases, the healthcare provider may need to consider more aggressive treatment strategies, such as the use of systemic corticosteroids or immunomodulatory agents, in addition to collaborating with specialists to address any underlying medical conditions.

Considerations in Special Populations

Diaper dermatitis may require unique considerations and adaptations in certain special populations, such as:

1. Premature infants: The delicate skin of premature infants may be more susceptible to diaper dermatitis, necessitating gentle skin care and close monitoring.
2. Individuals with incontinence: Adults or the elderly who experience incontinence may also develop diaper dermatitis, requiring tailored prevention and management strategies.
3. Individuals with physical or cognitive disabilities: Patients with limited mobility or cognitive impairments may require specialized caregiver support and adaptations to address their unique needs.

In these situations, healthcare providers should work closely with the patient, caregivers, and interdisciplinary teams to develop a comprehensive and personalized management plan that addresses the specific challenges and needs of the individual.

Conclusion

Diaper dermatitis is a common and often distressing form of irritant contact dermatitis that predominantly affects infants and toddlers. In this chapter, we have explored the underlying etiology of this skin condition, highlighting the key factors that contribute to its development, such as prolonged exposure to urine, feces, and other irritants, as well as the role of occlusion, friction, and microbial imbalances.

We have also discussed the various risk factors and predisposing conditions that can increase the likelihood of developing diaper dermatitis, including age, diarrhea, antibiotic use, and underlying skin disorders. Understanding these risk factors is crucial for healthcare providers and caregivers to implement targeted preventive measures and provide appropriate management strategies.

The chapter has delved into the characteristic clinical presentation of diaper dermatitis, outlining the diagnostic considerations that can help healthcare providers distinguish this condition from other skin disorders. Additionally, we have presented a comprehensive approach to the prevention and management of diaper dermatitis, emphasizing the importance of proper diapering and skin care techniques, the use of topical and systemic therapies, and the need to address any underlying medical conditions.

Recognizing the potential for complications and the unique considerations in special populations, we have highlighted the importance of vigilance, adaptability, and a collaborative approach to ensure the best possible outcomes for infants and toddlers affected by this troublesome skin condition.

By equipping healthcare providers and caregivers with the knowledge and strategies presented in this chapter, we aim to empower them to effectively prevent, identify, and manage diaper dermatitis, ultimately improving the quality of life for the affected children and their families.

CHAPTER 6

Dermatitis Herpetiformis

Dermatitis herpetiformis, also known as Duhring's disease, is a rare and chronic autoimmune skin condition that is closely associated with celiac disease. This unique form of dermatitis is characterized by intensely itchy, blistering rashes that can significantly impact an individual's quality of life. In this chapter, we will delve into the pathogenesis and genetic association of dermatitis herpetiformis, explore its clinical manifestations and diagnostic criteria, and discuss the latest advancements in the treatment and management of this complex skin disorder.

Understanding the Pathogenesis and Genetic Association

Dermatitis herpetiformis is an autoimmune disorder in which the body's immune system mistakenly attacks its own tissues, leading to the development of the characteristic skin lesions. The underlying mechanisms driving the pathogenesis of this condition are closely linked to celiac disease, a well-established autoimmune disorder affecting the small intestine.

Gluten-Induced Autoimmunity

At the core of dermatitis herpetiformis is an aberrant immune response to the ingestion of gluten, a protein found in wheat, barley, and rye. In individuals with dermatitis herpetiformis, the consumption of gluten triggers an autoimmune reaction, leading to the production of specific antibodies that target the skin and the small intestine.

The primary autoantibodies involved in dermatitis herpetiformis are directed against a protein called transglutaminase 3 (TG3), which is predominantly found in the skin. These autoantibodies, along with other immune complexes, accumulate in the skin and trigger an intense inflammatory response, resulting in the characteristic blistering and pruritic rash.

Genetic Predisposition

Dermatitis herpetiformis, like celiac disease, has a strong genetic component, with the majority of individuals with the condition carrying specific human leukocyte antigen (HLA) genotypes, primarily the HLA-DQ2 and HLA-DQ8 haplotypes.

These genetic variations play a crucial role in the presentation and development of the autoimmune response in dermatitis herpetiformis. The HLA-DQ2 and HLA-DQ8 molecules are involved in the presentation of gluten-derived peptides to T cells, which in turn triggers the production of the autoantibodies targeting TG3 and other skin components.

In addition to the HLA genotypes, other genetic factors, such as polymorphisms in genes related to immune system regulation, have also been associated with an increased risk of developing dermatitis herpetiformis. However, the exact genetic mechanisms underlying the pathogenesis of this condition are still being actively investigated.

Clinical Manifestations and Diagnosis

Dermatitis herpetiformis presents with a distinct set of clinical features that can help healthcare providers differentiate it from other skin disorders. Understanding the characteristic symptoms and the diagnostic approach is essential for ensuring timely and accurate management of this condition.

Clinical Presentation

The hallmark symptoms of dermatitis herpetiformis include:

1. Intensely itchy skin lesions: The primary manifestation of dermatitis herpetiformis is the development of intensely pruritic, small, fluid-filled blisters or vesicles.
2. Symmetrical distribution: The skin lesions typically appear in a symmetrical pattern, most commonly on the elbows, knees, back, and buttocks.
3. Herpetiform arrangement: The blisters and vesicles often cluster in a "herpetiform" (or "cluster of grapes") arrangement, which is a distinguishing feature of this condition.
4. Erythema and urticarial plaques: In addition to the blisters, the affected skin may also exhibit erythema (redness) and urticarial (hive-like) plaques.
5. Chronic and relapsing nature: Dermatitis herpetiformis is a chronic, relapsing condition, with periods of flare-ups and remission.

It is important to note that the skin lesions in dermatitis herpetiformis can sometimes resemble those seen in other blistering skin conditions, such as pemphigoid or linear IgA disease, making accurate diagnosis crucial.

Diagnostic Evaluation

The diagnosis of dermatitis herpetiformis typically involves a combination of clinical evaluation, serological testing, and histopathological analysis.

1. Medical history and physical examination: The healthcare provider will obtain a detailed medical history, focusing on the onset, distribution, and characteristics of the skin lesions. A thorough physical examination, including an assessment of the skin and any associated symptoms, is essential.

2. Serological testing: Blood tests can be used to detect the presence of specific autoantibodies, such as those directed against tissue transglutaminase (tTG) and epidermal transglutaminase (eTG), which are commonly elevated in individuals with dermatitis herpetiformis.

3. Skin biopsy and direct immunofluorescence: A skin biopsy, followed by direct immunofluorescence analysis, can provide definitive diagnostic confirmation. This technique allows for the detection of characteristic immunoglobulin A (IgA) deposits within the skin, which is a hallmark feature of dermatitis herpetiformis.

4. Intestinal biopsy: In some cases, a small intestinal biopsy may be performed to assess for the presence of villous atrophy, which is commonly associated with celiac disease and can help confirm the underlying gluten sensitivity.

By combining the clinical presentation, serological findings, and histopathological analysis, healthcare providers can accurately diagnose dermatitis herpetiformis and differentiate it from other similar skin conditions.

Treatment and Management Strategies

The management of dermatitis herpetiformis focuses on two primary goals: relieving the symptoms and addressing the underlying autoimmune mechanism driving the condition. A multifaceted approach, involving both pharmacological and dietary interventions, is typically employed to achieve these objectives.

Dietary Management

The cornerstone of dermatitis herpetiformis management is the adoption of a strict, lifelong gluten-free diet. This dietary intervention aims to eliminate the trigger for the autoimmune response, thereby reducing the production of the offending autoantibodies and alleviating the skin manifestations.

1. Gluten-free diet: Patients with dermatitis herpetiformis must adhere to a strict gluten-free diet, avoiding all foods containing wheat, barley, rye, and their derivatives. This may require significant lifestyle changes and close monitoring to ensure complete gluten elimination.

2. Dietary education and support: Healthcare providers should work closely with patients to provide comprehensive education on the gluten-free diet, including guidance on food selection, meal planning, and dining out. Ongoing support and monitoring are crucial to ensure the patient's adherence and nutritional adequacy.

3. Monitoring and follow-up: Regular follow-up visits and laboratory tests, such as periodic measurement of serum antibody levels, can help assess the patient's response to the gluten-free diet and guide any necessary adjustments.

Pharmacological Interventions

In addition to the dietary management, healthcare providers may also prescribe pharmacological therapies to alleviate the symptoms and facilitate the healing of the skin lesions.

1. Antipruritic agents: Medications with antipruritic (anti-itch) properties, such as antihistamines or topical corticosteroids, can be used to provide symptomatic relief and reduce the intensity of the itching.

2. Dapsone: Dapsone, an antimicrobial agent with anti-inflammatory properties, is considered the primary pharmacological treatment for dermatitis herpetiformis. Dapsone can effectively reduce the severity and accelerate the healing of the skin lesions, although it may have potential side effects that require close monitoring.

3. Systemic corticosteroids: In cases of severe or recalcitrant skin lesions, short-term use of systemic corticosteroids may be considered to quickly

control the inflammatory response and provide symptomatic relief.

4. Immunosuppressants: In patients with refractory or severe cases of dermatitis herpetiformis, healthcare providers may prescribe immunosuppressant medications, such as azathioprine or methotrexate, to modulate the underlying autoimmune response.

It is important to note that the use of pharmacological interventions, particularly dapsone and immunosuppressants, requires close monitoring and management of potential side effects by healthcare providers with experience in treating dermatitis herpetiformis.

Monitoring and Ongoing Care

Effective management of dermatitis herpetiformis involves not only the initial treatment but also long-term monitoring and care. Healthcare providers should establish a comprehensive follow-up plan to assess the patient's response to the gluten-free diet and any pharmacological therapies, as well as to monitor for the development of any complications or associated conditions.

1. Periodic assessments: Regular clinical evaluations, including a comprehensive skin examination and assessment of symptom control, are essential to ensure the ongoing management of dermatitis herpetiformis.

2. Laboratory monitoring: Periodic blood tests, such as measuring serum antibody levels and monitoring for any nutritional deficiencies, can help guide the management approach and detect any changes in the patient's condition.

3. Screening for associated conditions: Individuals with dermatitis herpetiformis have an increased risk of developing other autoimmune or gastrointestinal conditions, such as celiac disease, thyroid disorders, or other malabsorption syndromes. Routine screening and vigilance for these

associated conditions are crucial.

4. Multidisciplinary collaboration: In some cases, a multidisciplinary approach, involving healthcare providers from various specialties (e.g., dermatology, gastroenterology, nutrition), may be necessary to provide comprehensive care and address the complex needs of patients with dermatitis herpetiformis.

By implementing a comprehensive and collaborative approach to the ongoing management of dermatitis herpetiformis, healthcare providers can help patients achieve better control over their condition, minimize the risk of complications, and improve their overall quality of life.

Prognosis and Complications

The prognosis for individuals with dermatitis herpetiformis is generally favorable, particularly when the condition is properly managed with a strict gluten-free diet and appropriate pharmacological interventions. However, it is important to be aware of the potential complications and long-term considerations associated with this condition.

Prognosis

With strict adherence to a gluten-free diet, the majority of patients with dermatitis herpetiformis can achieve significant improvement or complete remission of their skin lesions. The time required to achieve this response can vary, with some patients experiencing a more rapid resolution of symptoms, while others may require a longer period of dietary adaptation and treatment.

In cases where patients strictly adhere to the gluten-free diet, the long-term prognosis is generally favorable, with a reduced risk of complications and a good quality of life. However, it is important to note that in a small percentage of patients, the skin lesions may persist or recur despite a gluten-free diet, necessitating the use of additional pharmacological therapies.

Potential Complications

While the prognosis for dermatitis herpetiformis is generally good, there are several potential complications and associated conditions that healthcare providers should be aware of:

1. Celiac disease: As dermatitis herpetiformis is closely linked to celiac disease, individuals with this skin condition have an increased risk of developing or already having underlying celiac disease. Careful monitoring and management of the gastrointestinal aspects of the condition are crucial.

2. Malabsorption and nutritional deficiencies: The gluten-induced damage to the small intestine in celiac disease can lead to malabsorption of essential nutrients, such as iron, folate, and vitamin B12. Healthcare providers should routinely screen for and address any nutritional deficiencies.

3. Autoimmune thyroid disorders: Individuals with dermatitis herpetiformis have an elevated risk of developing autoimmune thyroid conditions, such as Hashimoto's thyroiditis or Graves' disease. Regular screening and monitoring for thyroid dysfunction are recommended.

4. Lymphoproliferative disorders: There is a small increased risk of developing certain types of lymphoma, particularly in patients with long-standing, poorly controlled celiac disease or dermatitis herpetiformis. Vigilance and appropriate screening are necessary.

5. Renal complications: In rare cases, dermatitis herpetiformis may be associated with the deposition of immune complexes in the kidneys, leading to glomerulonephritis or other renal complications. Regular monitoring of kidney function is advised.

By being aware of these potential complications and implementing appropriate screening and management strategies, healthcare providers can help optimize the long-term outcomes for individuals with dermatitis herpetiformis and minimize the risk of associated health issues.

Conclusion

Dermatitis herpetiformis is a rare and complex autoimmune skin condition that is closely linked to celiac disease. In this chapter, we have delved into the pathogenesis of this condition, highlighting the pivotal role of gluten-induced autoimmunity and the strong genetic predisposition associated with specific HLA genotypes.

We have explored the characteristic clinical manifestations of dermatitis herpetiformis, including the intense itching, blistering rash, and herpetiform distribution of the skin lesions. Understanding the diagnostic approach, which involves a combination of clinical evaluation, serological testing, and histopathological analysis, is crucial for ensuring timely and accurate diagnosis.

The management of dermatitis herpetiformis centers around a two-pronged approach: dietary intervention with a strict gluten-free diet and the use of pharmacological therapies, such as dapsone and immunosuppressants, to alleviate symptoms and modulate the underlying autoimmune response. The importance of ongoing monitoring, screening for associated conditions, and a collaborative, multidisciplinary approach to patient care has also been emphasized.

By equipping healthcare providers with a comprehensive understanding of dermatitis herpetiformis, this chapter aims to empower them to deliver effective and personalized care to individuals living with this rare and challenging skin condition. The insights gained here will serve as a valuable foundation for the holistic management of this disorder, ultimately improving the quality of life for those affected.

CHAPTER 7

Nummular Dermatitis

Nummular dermatitis, also known as nummular eczema or discoid eczema, is a distinct form of dermatitis characterized by the development of circular or coin-shaped skin lesions. This chronic and often perplexing condition can cause significant discomfort and distress for those affected. In this chapter, we will explore the epidemiology and underlying causes of nummular dermatitis, delve into its clinical characteristics and diagnostic criteria, and discuss the various management strategies employed to alleviate the symptoms and improve the overall quality of life for patients.

Epidemiology and Causes of Nummular Dermatitis

Nummular dermatitis is considered a relatively uncommon form of dermatitis, but its true prevalence is not well-established due to potential underdiagnosis and variations in reporting across different regions and populations. However, studies suggest that it can affect individuals of all ages, with a higher incidence observed in older adults.

Epidemiology

Nummular dermatitis can occur at any age, but it is more commonly reported in adults, particularly those between the ages of 55 and 65. The condition appears to have a slightly higher prevalence in males compared to females, though the exact gender distribution may vary across different studies.

Geographical and seasonal factors may also play a role in the incidence of nummular dermatitis, with some studies suggesting a higher prevalence in colder, drier climates and during the winter months. This seasonal variation may be attributed to the exacerbating effect of environmental factors, such as low humidity and increased exposure to irritants, on the skin's barrier function.

Underlying Causes and Predisposing Factors

The exact etiology of nummular dermatitis is not fully understood, but it is believed to be multifactorial, involving a complex interplay of various genetic, environmental, and physiological factors.

Dry Skin and Skin Barrier Dysfunction

One of the primary contributors to the development of nummular dermatitis is the presence of inherently dry skin and impaired skin barrier function. Individuals with a history of atopic dermatitis or other skin conditions associated with xerosis (dry skin) may be more predisposed to developing nummular dermatitis.

The disruption of the skin's barrier function, often due to environmental factors, such as low humidity or excessive bathing, can lead to increased transepidermal water loss and the subsequent development of the characteristic coin-shaped skin lesions.

Underlying Medical Conditions

In some cases, nummular dermatitis may be associated with or exacerbated by underlying medical conditions, including:

1. Atopic dermatitis: Individuals with a history of atopic dermatitis are at

an increased risk of developing nummular dermatitis.

2. Allergic contact dermatitis: Exposure to contact allergens, such as metals or chemicals, can trigger the development of nummular dermatitis in susceptible individuals.

3. Seborrheic dermatitis: The presence of seborrheic dermatitis in certain body areas may predispose individuals to the development of nummular lesions.

4. Xerosis: Conditions that lead to generalized dry skin, such as hypothyroidism or Sjögren's syndrome, can increase the risk of nummular dermatitis.

Mechanical Factors and Skin Injuries

Minor skin injuries, such as bug bites, scratches, or burns, can sometimes trigger the formation of nummular lesions in individuals with a predisposition to the condition. The skin's response to these minor traumas may contribute to the development of the characteristic coin-shaped plaques.

Genetic Factors

While the genetic component of nummular dermatitis is not as well-established as in other forms of dermatitis, such as atopic dermatitis, some studies have suggested a potential role of genetic factors in the predisposition to this condition. However, more research is needed to fully elucidate the genetic underpinnings of nummular dermatitis.

Overall, the multifactorial nature of nummular dermatitis, with its complex interplay of skin barrier dysfunction, underlying medical conditions, and environmental triggers, underscores the importance of a comprehensive approach to its management and prevention.

Clinical Characteristics and Diagnostic Criteria

Nummular dermatitis presents with a distinctive set of clinical features that can help healthcare providers differentiate it from other skin conditions. Understanding the characteristic lesions and diagnostic considerations is crucial for accurate diagnosis and appropriate management.

Clinical Presentation

The hallmark feature of nummular dermatitis is the development of circular or coin-shaped skin lesions, which are the primary basis for the condition's name. These lesions typically exhibit the following characteristics:

1. Coin-shaped appearance: The skin lesions are well-defined, circular or oval-shaped, and often range in size from a few millimeters to several centimeters in diameter.
2. Raised or plaque-like structure: The lesions have a slightly raised, plaque-like appearance, with a distinct border.
3. Erythema and scaling: The skin within the lesions typically appears red and may exhibit varying degrees of scaling, flakiness, or crusting.
4. Pruritus: Patients with nummular dermatitis often experience moderate to severe itching, which can significantly impact their quality of life.
5. Distribution: The lesions most commonly appear on the extremities, particularly the lower legs, but can also affect other areas of the body, such as the trunk or hands.
6. Chronic and recurrent nature: Nummular dermatitis is a chronic condition, with periods of flare-ups and remission. Patients may experience recurrent episodes of the characteristic skin lesions over time.

Diagnostic Criteria and Evaluation

Diagnosing nummular dermatitis typically involves a comprehensive clinical evaluation, including a thorough medical history and physical examination. Healthcare providers may use the following diagnostic criteria to identify and confirm the condition:

1. Presence of coin-shaped or circular skin lesions
2. Characteristic morphology, including erythema, scaling, and a raised, plaque-like appearance
3. Pruritus associated with the skin lesions
4. Chronic or recurrent nature of the condition
5. Exclusion of other skin conditions that may present with similar features, such as psoriasis or tinea corporis

In some cases, healthcare providers may perform additional diagnostic tests, such as:

1. Skin biopsy: A skin biopsy can help rule out other skin conditions and provide confirmatory histopathological evidence of nummular dermatitis.
2. Patch testing: If allergic contact dermatitis is suspected as a contributing factor, patch testing may be performed to identify any relevant allergens.
3. Laboratory tests: Routine blood tests or specific laboratory investigations may be ordered to assess for any underlying medical conditions that may be associated with nummular dermatitis.

By combining the clinical presentation, patient history, and, if necessary, ancillary diagnostic tests, healthcare providers can accurately diagnose nummular dermatitis and differentiate it from other similar skin conditions.

Management and Treatment Strategies

The management of nummular dermatitis typically involves a multifaceted approach, focusing on addressing the underlying causes, relieving the symptoms, and preventing the recurrence of the characteristic skin lesions. Healthcare providers may employ a combination of topical therapies, systemic interventions, and lifestyle modifications to achieve optimal outcomes for patients.

Topical Treatments

The primary line of treatment for nummular dermatitis involves the use of topical therapies to manage the skin lesions and alleviate the associated symptoms.

1. Emollients and moisturizers: Maintaining the skin's hydration and barrier function is crucial in the management of nummular dermatitis. Healthcare providers may recommend the use of fragrance-free, hypoallergenic emollients and moisturizers to help restore the skin's protective layer.

2. Topical corticosteroids: Low- to moderate-potency topical corticosteroids can be used to reduce inflammation, itching, and the severity of the skin lesions. These should be applied judiciously and under the close supervision of a healthcare provider.

3. Calcineurin inhibitors: In cases where topical corticosteroids are contraindicated or ineffective, topical calcineurin inhibitors, such as tacrolimus or pimecrolimus, may be prescribed to modulate the immune response and alleviate the skin lesions.

4. Topical antimicrobials: If secondary bacterial or fungal infections are present, the healthcare provider may recommend the use of topical antimicrobial agents to manage the infection and prevent further complications.

Systemic Interventions

In more severe or widespread cases of nummular dermatitis, the healthcare provider may consider the use of systemic therapies to supplement the topical treatment approach.

1. Oral antihistamines: Oral antihistamines can be helpful in managing the

associated pruritus and providing symptomatic relief.

2. Oral corticosteroids: In cases of severe or recalcitrant nummular dermatitis, a short course of oral corticosteroids may be prescribed to quickly control the inflammation and promote healing.

3. Immunosuppressants: For patients with chronic, treatment-resistant nummular dermatitis, the healthcare provider may consider the use of oral or injectable immunosuppressant medications, such as methotrexate or dupilumab, to modulate the underlying immune response.

Phototherapy and Photochemotherapy

In some instances, healthcare providers may recommend the use of phototherapy or photochemotherapy as an adjunct to the treatment of nummular dermatitis.

1. Narrow-band UVB phototherapy: This targeted form of ultraviolet light therapy can help reduce inflammation and promote the healing of the skin lesions.

2. PUVA (psoralen plus UVA) therapy: The combination of a photosensitizing agent (psoralen) and UVA light exposure can be effective in the management of nummular dermatitis, particularly in cases where other treatments have been unsuccessful.

Addressing Underlying Conditions

Given the potential association between nummular dermatitis and various underlying medical conditions, healthcare providers should carefully evaluate and address any contributing factors that may be exacerbating the patient's skin condition.

1. Treating atopic dermatitis or contact dermatitis: Addressing the underlying atopic or contact dermatitis can help improve the overall management

of nummular dermatitis.

2. Addressing dry skin and skin barrier dysfunction: Implementing measures to improve skin hydration and barrier function, such as the use of emollients and avoidance of irritants, can be beneficial.

3. Managing underlying medical conditions: If nummular dermatitis is associated with conditions like hypothyroidism or Sjögren's syndrome, addressing the underlying disorder may help alleviate the skin manifestations.

Lifestyle Modifications and Prevention

In addition to the medical treatments, healthcare providers should also emphasize the importance of lifestyle modifications and preventive measures to help manage nummular dermatitis and reduce the risk of recurrence.

1. Skin care and bathing routines: Recommending the use of gentle, fragrance-free cleansers and the adoption of a consistent moisturizing routine can help maintain the skin's barrier function.

2. Avoidance of irritants: Identifying and minimizing exposure to potential skin irritants, such as harsh detergents, chemicals, or extreme environmental conditions, can help prevent the development or exacerbation of nummular dermatitis.

3. Stress management: Incorporating stress-reducing techniques, such as relaxation exercises, meditation, or counseling, may help alleviate the impact of stress on the condition.

4. Proactive monitoring: Regular follow-up with the healthcare provider, including monitoring for any underlying medical conditions, can help detect and address flare-ups or complications in a timely manner.

By incorporating a comprehensive, multifaceted approach to the management of nummular dermatitis, healthcare providers can work collaboratively with patients to achieve better control over the condition, alleviate the associated symptoms, and improve the overall quality of life.

Prognosis and Considerations

The prognosis for individuals with nummular dermatitis can vary depending on the severity of the condition, the underlying factors, and the patient's response to the prescribed treatments. While the condition is often chronic and relapsing, proper management can significantly improve the long-term outcomes and quality of life for those affected.

Prognosis

The overall prognosis for nummular dermatitis is generally favorable, with most patients able to achieve good control of their skin condition through a combination of topical therapies, systemic interventions, and lifestyle modifications. However, the chronic and recurrent nature of the condition means that many individuals may experience periodic flare-ups and require ongoing management.

In cases where the underlying causes, such as atopic dermatitis or contact dermatitis, can be effectively addressed, the prognosis is typically better, with the potential for longer periods of remission. Conversely, patients with more severe or treatment-resistant nummular dermatitis may require more intensive and prolonged management, with a higher risk of persistent or recurrent skin lesions.

Considerations and Comorbidities

While nummular dermatitis is primarily a skin condition, healthcare providers should be mindful of the potential associations and comorbidities that may accompany this disorder.

1. Atopic dermatitis: Individuals with a history of atopic dermatitis are at an

increased risk of developing nummular dermatitis, and the two conditions may coexist, requiring a coordinated management approach.

2. Allergic contact dermatitis: In some cases, nummular dermatitis may be triggered or exacerbated by exposure to contact allergens, necessitating the identification and avoidance of the offending agent(s).

3. Dry skin and xerosis: The presence of inherently dry skin and impaired skin barrier function can contribute to the development and recurrence of nummular dermatitis, underscoring the importance of comprehensive skin care and hydration.

4. Underlying medical conditions: As mentioned earlier, nummular dermatitis may be associated with or exacerbated by various medical conditions, such as hypothyroidism or Sjögren's syndrome. Careful evaluation and management of these underlying disorders are crucial.

By recognizing the potential comorbidities and considering the unique aspects of each patient's presentation, healthcare providers can develop a personalized management plan that addresses the multifaceted nature of nummular dermatitis and optimizes the long-term outcomes for individuals living with this chronic skin condition.

Conclusion

Nummular dermatitis is a distinctive form of dermatitis characterized by the development of circular or coin-shaped skin lesions. In this chapter, we have explored the epidemiological and etiological factors contributing to the development of this condition, highlighting the role of dry skin, underlying medical conditions, and environmental triggers in the pathogenesis of nummular dermatitis.

We have delved into the characteristic clinical presentation of nummular dermatitis, including the distinctive morphology of the skin lesions, the associated pruritus, and the chronic, recurrent nature of the condition. Understanding the diagnostic criteria and the various evaluation techniques employed by healthcare providers is crucial for ensuring accurate diagnosis and appropriate management.

The comprehensive management strategies for nummular dermatitis involve a combination of topical therapies, systemic interventions, phototherapy, and targeted approaches to address any underlying medical conditions or triggers. Emphasizing the importance of lifestyle modifications and preventive measures further reinforces the holistic approach to the care of individuals with this chronic skin disorder.

By equipping healthcare providers with a thorough understanding of nummular dermatitis, this chapter aims to empower them to deliver effective and personalized care to patients, ultimately improving the quality of life for those affected by this perplexing and often challenging skin condition. The insights gained here will serve as a valuable foundation as we continue our exploration of the diverse forms of dermatitis.

CHAPTER 8

Stasis Dermatitis

Stasis dermatitis, also known as gravitational dermatitis or venous eczema, is a chronic and often recurrent skin condition that is closely associated with underlying venous insufficiency and poor circulation. This type of dermatitis can lead to significant discomfort, secondary complications, and a substantial impact on an individual's quality of life. In this chapter, we will delve into the pathophysiology and underlying conditions that contribute to the development of stasis dermatitis, explore its clinical presentation and diagnostic considerations, and discuss the comprehensive management strategies employed to alleviate the symptoms and prevent the progression of this troublesome skin disorder.

Understanding the Pathophysiology and Underlying Conditions

The development of stasis dermatitis is primarily driven by the presence of underlying venous insufficiency, a condition in which the veins in the lower extremities are unable to effectively pump blood back to the heart, leading to venous stasis and the accumulation of fluid in the skin and surrounding tissues.

Pathophysiology of Stasis Dermatitis

The key pathophysiological mechanisms underlying stasis dermatitis include:

1. Venous insufficiency: Impaired venous function, often due to valvular dysfunction or venous obstruction, leads to the pooling of blood and fluid in the lower extremities.

2. Increased hydrostatic pressure: The accumulation of fluid in the skin and subcutaneous tissues, as a result of venous insufficiency, increases the hydrostatic pressure in the affected areas.

3. Inflammation and skin changes: The elevated hydrostatic pressure and impaired circulation lead to inflammation, increased capillary permeability, and subsequent changes in the skin, including edema, pigmentation, and the development of characteristic skin lesions.

4. Skin barrier dysfunction: The chronic inflammation and alterations in the skin's structure can contribute to a compromised skin barrier, further exacerbating the condition and increasing the risk of secondary infections.

Underlying Conditions and Risk Factors

The development of stasis dermatitis is closely linked to various underlying medical conditions and risk factors that contribute to the impairment of venous function and the subsequent development of the skin disorder.

1. Venous insufficiency: This is the primary underlying condition associated with stasis dermatitis. Conditions that can lead to venous insufficiency include:
   - Deep vein thrombosis (DVT)
   - Chronic venous insufficiency (CVI)
   - Varicose veins
   - Venous valve dysfunction

2. Cardiovascular and circulatory disorders:
   - Congestive heart failure
   - Peripheral artery disease

- Diabetes mellitus with associated vascular complications

3. Obesity and sedentary lifestyle:
- Excess weight can increase the risk of venous insufficiency and poor circulation.
- Lack of physical activity can contribute to the development of venous stasis.

4. Advanced age:
- The prevalence of venous insufficiency and associated skin changes increases with age.

5. Previous history of leg injuries or trauma:
- Damage to the veins or lymphatic system can impair circulation and lead to the development of stasis dermatitis.

By understanding the pathophysiological mechanisms and the underlying conditions that predispose individuals to stasis dermatitis, healthcare providers can develop a comprehensive approach to the diagnosis, management, and prevention of this skin disorder.

Clinical Presentation and Diagnostic Considerations

Stasis dermatitis presents with a characteristic set of clinical features that can help healthcare providers differentiate it from other skin conditions. Recognizing the distinctive signs and symptoms is crucial for accurate diagnosis and appropriate management.

Clinical Characteristics
The hallmark features of stasis dermatitis include:

1. Erythema and edema: The affected skin, typically on the lower extrem-

ities, appears red and swollen due to the accumulation of fluid and inflammation.

2. Pigmentation changes: The skin may exhibit brown or reddish-brown discoloration, often referred to as "stasis pigmentation," due to the deposition of hemosiderin (a breakdown product of red blood cells).

3. Scaling and lichenification: The skin may develop a thickened, leathery appearance (lichenification) and exhibit flaky, scaly patches.

4. Pruritus and discomfort: Patients with stasis dermatitis often experience moderate to severe itching, as well as a burning or aching sensation in the affected areas.

5. Ulceration and crusting: In more advanced cases, the skin may develop open sores or ulcers, which can be prone to crusting and secondary infections.

6. Unilateral or bilateral distribution: The skin lesions are typically localized to the lower extremities, with a unilateral or bilateral involvement depending on the underlying venous insufficiency.

Diagnostic Evaluation

Diagnosing stasis dermatitis involves a comprehensive clinical assessment, including a thorough medical history and physical examination, as well as the consideration of potential underlying conditions.

1. Medical history: Healthcare providers will gather information about the patient's symptoms, the onset and progression of the skin lesions, and any underlying medical conditions, such as venous insufficiency, cardiovascular disorders, or previous leg injuries.

2. Physical examination: A detailed examination of the affected skin, including an assessment of the appearance, distribution, and associated symptoms, is crucial for identifying the characteristic features of stasis dermatitis.

3. Diagnostic tests:

- Vascular assessment: Doppler ultrasonography or other imaging techniques may be employed to evaluate the underlying venous function and identify any evidence of venous insufficiency.

- Skin biopsy: In some cases, a skin biopsy may be performed to rule out other skin conditions or confirm the diagnosis of stasis dermatitis.

- Laboratory tests: Routine blood tests, such as complete blood count and metabolic panel, may be ordered to assess for any underlying medical conditions that could contribute to the development of stasis dermatitis.

By combining the clinical presentation, patient history, and, if necessary, diagnostic test results, healthcare providers can accurately diagnose stasis dermatitis and differentiate it from other skin disorders, such as contact dermatitis, psoriasis, or venous ulcers.

Stages and Progression of Stasis Dermatitis

Stasis dermatitis is a progressive condition that can evolve through various stages, with the severity and extent of the skin lesions often correlating with the underlying venous insufficiency and associated complications.

Early Stages

In the early stages of stasis dermatitis, the affected skin may exhibit only mild erythema, edema, and a slight discoloration. Patients may experience occasional pruritus or a burning sensation, but the skin lesions are typically limited in extent and severity.

Intermediate Stages

As the condition progresses, the skin changes become more pronounced, with the development of more extensive erythema, scaling, and lichenification. The pigmentation changes, such as the characteristic brown or reddish-brown discoloration, become more evident. Pruritus and discomfort may become more troublesome for the patient during this stage.

Advanced Stages

In the advanced stages of stasis dermatitis, the skin lesions may become more severe, with the potential development of ulcerations, crusting, and an increased risk of secondary infections. The underlying venous insufficiency and associated complications, such as edema and poor circulation, are often more pronounced, contributing to the worsening of the skin condition.

Progression and Complications

The progression of stasis dermatitis is closely tied to the underlying venous insufficiency and the associated cardiovascular or circulatory disorders. Uncontrolled or worsening venous dysfunction can lead to the following complications:

1. Venous ulceration: The breakdown of the skin and underlying tissues can result in the formation of painful, slow-healing venous ulcers.
2. Cellulitis and skin infections: The compromised skin barrier and poor circulation increase the risk of secondary bacterial or fungal infections, which can further exacerbate the skin condition.
3. Lymphedema: Chronic venous insufficiency can lead to the accumulation of lymphatic fluid, resulting in swelling and the development of lymphedema.
4. Reduced mobility and quality of life: The pain, discomfort, and disfigurement associated with advanced stasis dermatitis can significantly impact an individual's physical and emotional well-being, limiting their mobility and quality of life.

Recognizing the stages of stasis dermatitis and being vigilant for potential complications is crucial for healthcare providers to implement appropriate management strategies and prevent the progression of the condition.

Management and Treatment Strategies

The management of stasis dermatitis typically involves a multi-pronged approach, focusing on addressing the underlying venous insufficiency, managing the skin lesions, and preventing the development of complications. Healthcare providers may employ a combination of medical, surgical, and lifestyle-based interventions to achieve optimal outcomes for patients.

Addressing Venous Insufficiency

The primary goal in the management of stasis dermatitis is to address the underlying venous dysfunction and improve the circulatory status of the affected limb(s).

1. Compression therapy: The use of compression stockings or bandages can help improve venous return, reduce edema, and mitigate the progression of venous insufficiency.
2. Leg elevation: Elevating the affected limb(s) above the level of the heart can help promote venous return and reduce fluid accumulation.
3. Pharmacological interventions: Certain medications, such as venoactive drugs or anticoagulants, may be prescribed to improve venous function and prevent the complications of venous insufficiency.
4. Surgical interventions: In cases of severe or refractory venous insufficiency, healthcare providers may consider surgical options, such as vein stripping, endovenous ablation, or valve repair, to restore proper venous function.

Topical Treatments for Skin Lesions

Alongside the management of the underlying venous condition, healthcare providers will also focus on addressing the skin lesions associated with stasis dermatitis.

1. Emollients and moisturizers: The use of fragrance-free, hypoallergenic

moisturizers can help hydrate the skin and improve the skin barrier function.

2. Topical corticosteroids: Low- to medium-potency topical corticosteroids can be used to reduce inflammation and provide symptomatic relief for the pruritus and discomfort.
3. Topical antibiotics or antifungals: In the presence of secondary skin infections, the healthcare provider may prescribe topical antimicrobial agents to manage the infection and prevent further complications.
4. Keratolytic agents: Topical products containing ingredients like urea or salicylic acid can help promote the shedding of thickened, scaly skin and improve the appearance of the lesions.

Systemic Interventions

In more severe or refractory cases of stasis dermatitis, the healthcare provider may consider the use of systemic therapies to supplement the topical and compression-based treatments.

1. Oral antihistamines: Oral antihistamines can be helpful in managing the associated pruritus and providing symptomatic relief.
2. Oral corticosteroids: A short course of oral corticosteroids may be prescribed to quickly control severe inflammation and promote healing, particularly in cases with extensive skin involvement.
3. Immunosuppressants: For patients with chronic, treatment-resistant stasis dermatitis, the healthcare provider may consider the use of oral or injectable immunosuppressant medications, such as methotrexate or dupilumab, to modulate the underlying immune response.

Wound Care and Management of Complications

In cases where stasis dermatitis has progressed to the development of skin ulcers or other complications, the healthcare provider will focus on comprehensive wound care and the prevention of further complications.

1. Wound dressings: The use of appropriate wound dressings, such as hydrocolloids, hydrogels, or foam dressings, can help promote wound healing and prevent infection.
2. Debridement: Removal of devitalized or necrotic tissue through debridement can facilitate the healing process and reduce the risk of infection.
3. Antimicrobial therapy: Topical or systemic antimicrobial agents may be necessary to manage any secondary infections and prevent their spread.
4. Negative pressure wound therapy: In some cases, the use of negative pressure wound therapy (NPWT) can help accelerate the healing of chronic venous ulcers.

Lifestyle Modifications and Prevention

In addition to the medical and surgical interventions, healthcare providers should also emphasize the importance of lifestyle modifications and preventive measures to help manage stasis dermatitis and reduce the risk of recurrence or complications.

1. Weight management: Maintaining a healthy body weight can help improve venous function and reduce the risk of venous insufficiency.
2. Physical activity: Regular exercise, such as walking or leg exercises, can help improve circulation and venous return.
3. Skin care and hygiene: Adopting a consistent skin care routine, including the use of gentle cleansers and moisturizers, can help maintain the skin's barrier function and prevent further irritation.
4. Compression stockings: Wearing compression stockings or socks can help improve venous return and reduce the risk of edema and ulceration.
5. Regular follow-up: Ongoing monitoring and management of the under-

lying venous condition, as well as the skin lesions, are crucial to prevent the progression of stasis dermatitis and associated complications.

By employing a comprehensive, multi-faceted approach to the management of stasis dermatitis, healthcare providers can work collaboratively with patients to achieve better control over the condition, prevent the development of complications, and improve the overall quality of life for those affected by this challenging skin disorder.

Prognosis and Considerations

The prognosis for individuals with stasis dermatitis can vary depending on the severity of the underlying venous insufficiency, the extent and progression of the skin lesions, and the patient's response to the prescribed treatments. While stasis dermatitis is a chronic condition, appropriate management and addressing the underlying causes can significantly improve the long-term outcomes and quality of life for those affected.

Prognosis

The prognosis for stasis dermatitis is generally favorable when the underlying venous insufficiency is effectively managed and the skin lesions are appropriately treated. With a combination of compression therapy, appropriate medical and surgical interventions, and lifestyle modifications, many patients can achieve good control over their skin condition and prevent the progression of complications.

However, in cases where the venous dysfunction is severe or refractory to treatment, the prognosis may be more guarded. Persistent or recurrent skin lesions, the development of venous ulcers, and the increased risk of secondary infections can all contribute to a poorer long-term outlook.

Considerations and Comorbidities

Healthcare providers should be mindful of the potential comorbidities and associated conditions that may accompany stasis dermatitis, as these can have a significant impact on the patient's overall health and the management of the skin disorder.

1. Cardiovascular and circulatory disorders: Conditions such as congestive heart failure, peripheral artery disease, and diabetes mellitus can contribute to the development and progression of venous insufficiency and stasis dermatitis.

2. Obesity and sedentary lifestyle: Excess weight and physical inactivity can increase the risk of venous dysfunction and the associated skin changes.

3. Lymphedema: Chronic venous insufficiency can lead to the development of lymphedema, which may further exacerbate the skin condition and increase the risk of complications.

4. Skin infections and ulceration: The compromised skin barrier and poor circulation associated with stasis dermatitis can predispose individuals to the development of secondary skin infections and the formation of chronic, slow-healing venous ulcers.

5. Psychosocial impact: The visible skin lesions, discomfort, and associated limitations in mobility can have a significant impact on an individual's emotional well-being, self-esteem, and overall quality of life.

By recognizing these potential comorbidities and addressing the multifaceted aspects of stasis dermatitis, healthcare providers can develop a comprehensive management plan that optimizes the long-term outcomes and enhances the quality of life for individuals living with this chronic skin condition.

Conclusion

Stasis dermatitis is a chronic and often recurrent skin disorder that is closely associated with underlying venous insufficiency and poor circulation in the lower extremities. In this chapter, we have explored the pathophysiological mechanisms and the various underlying conditions that contribute to the development of this skin condition, highlighting the pivotal role of impaired venous function and the subsequent changes in the skin.

We have delved into the characteristic clinical presentation of stasis dermatitis, including the erythema, edema, pigmentation changes, and the potential for the development of ulcerations and secondary infections. Understanding the diagnostic approach, which involves a comprehensive assessment of the patient's medical history, physical examination, and relevant diagnostic tests, is crucial for accurate diagnosis and appropriate management.

The management of stasis dermatitis encompasses a multi-pronged strategy, focusing on addressing the underlying venous insufficiency through various medical, surgical, and lifestyle-based interventions, while also addressing the skin lesions through topical and systemic therapies. The importance of wound care and the prevention of complications, such as venous ulcers and skin infections, has also been emphasized.

By equipping healthcare providers with a thorough understanding of stasis dermatitis, this chapter aims to empower them to deliver effective and personalized care to patients, ultimately improving the quality of life for those affected by this challenging skin condition. The insights gained here will serve as a valuable foundation as we continue our exploration of the diverse forms of dermatitis.

CHAPTER 9

Perioral Dermatitis

Perioral dermatitis is a distinct form of facial dermatitis that primarily affects the skin around the mouth, nose, and chin area. This condition is characterized by the development of a red, scaly rash that can be both cosmetically and psychologically distressing for those affected. In this chapter, we will delve into the etiology and predisposing factors associated with perioral dermatitis, explore its clinical features and diagnostic criteria, and discuss the various management strategies employed to alleviate the symptoms and prevent the recurrence of this challenging skin disorder.

Understanding the Etiology and Predisposing Factors

The exact cause of perioral dermatitis is not fully understood, but it is believed to be a multifactorial condition, with a complex interplay of various contributing factors, including:

Topical Corticosteroid Use

One of the primary triggers for perioral dermatitis is the prolonged or inappropriate use of topical corticosteroids on the face. Repeated application of these potent anti-inflammatory agents can lead to a disruption of the skin's barrier function and an alteration in the skin's microbiome, ultimately contributing to the development of the characteristic rash.

It is important to note that perioral dermatitis is not limited to individuals who have used topical corticosteroids on their face, and the condition can also occur in those who have not had any prior exposure to these medications.

Cosmetic and Personal Care Products

The use of certain cosmetic and personal care products, particularly those containing irritants or occlusive ingredients, can also play a role in the development of perioral dermatitis. The skin around the mouth and nose is particularly susceptible to the effects of these products, which can disrupt the skin's barrier and lead to an inflammatory response.

Examples of problematic ingredients may include fragrances, preservatives, and occlusive agents, such as petrolatum or dimethicone. The overuse or improper application of these products can contribute to the onset of perioral dermatitis.

Hormonal Factors

Hormonal fluctuations and imbalances have also been implicated as potential contributing factors in the development of perioral dermatitis. The condition is more commonly observed in women, particularly during periods of hormonal changes, such as pregnancy, the postpartum period, or menopause.

The precise mechanisms by which hormonal factors may influence the development of perioral dermatitis are not fully understood, but it is believed that the changes in the skin's sebum production and immune responses may play a role.

Structural and Anatomical Factors

The unique anatomical and structural features of the skin around the mouth and nose may also predispose individuals to the development of perioral dermatitis. This area of the face is rich in sebaceous glands and has a higher density of hair follicles, which can contribute to the accumulation of sebum and the growth of microorganisms, potentially triggering an inflammatory response.

Additionally, the constant movement and exposure to environmental factors, such as food, saliva, and temperature changes, in the perioral region may further exacerbate the condition.

Genetic and Immunological Factors

While the genetic and immunological underpinnings of perioral dermatitis are not as well-established as in other forms of dermatitis, such as atopic dermatitis, there is some evidence suggesting a potential role of these factors in the predisposition to the condition.

Certain genetic variations or polymorphisms may influence the skin's barrier function, immune responses, or the susceptibility to environmental triggers, contributing to the development of perioral dermatitis in certain individuals.

Overall, the etiology of perioral dermatitis is multifactorial, with the interplay of various factors, including topical corticosteroid use, cosmetic products, hormonal influences, and structural/anatomical characteristics, contributing to the onset and manifestation of this skin disorder.

Clinical Presentation and Diagnostic Criteria

Perioral dermatitis presents with a distinctive set of clinical features that can help healthcare providers differentiate it from other skin conditions affecting the facial area. Understanding the characteristic appearance and distribution of the skin lesions is crucial for accurate diagnosis and appropriate management.

Clinical Characteristics

The hallmark features of perioral dermatitis include:

1. Erythema and papules: The primary manifestation of perioral dermatitis is the development of a red, inflamed rash around the mouth, often with the presence of small, raised bumps (papules).
2. Perifollicular distribution: The skin lesions typically exhibit a perifollicular distribution, meaning they are centered around the hair follicles in the affected area.
3. Scaling and dryness: The skin may appear scaly, flaky, or dry, with a rough or uneven texture.
4. Localized distribution: The rash is usually confined to the skin immediately surrounding the mouth, with the potential for extension to the nasolabial folds, chin, and cheeks.
5. Sparing of the vermilion border: Interestingly, the red, inflamed skin often spares the vermilion border (the junction between the lip and the skin).
6. Absence of comedones: Unlike acne, perioral dermatitis does not typically present with blackheads or whiteheads.

Diagnostic Criteria

Diagnosing perioral dermatitis typically involves a comprehensive clinical evaluation and assessment, as well as the consideration of the patient's medical history and potential contributing factors.

Healthcare providers may use the following diagnostic criteria to identify and confirm the presence of perioral dermatitis:

1. Presence of a red, scaly rash around the mouth, with a perifollicular distribution
2. Absence of comedones or other acne-like lesions
3. Sparing of the vermilion border of the lips
4. History of topical corticosteroid use or exposure to other potential triggers, such as cosmetic products

5. Exclusion of other skin conditions that may present with similar facial rashes, such as seborrheic dermatitis, contact dermatitis, or rosacea

In some cases, healthcare providers may perform additional diagnostic tests, such as skin biopsies or patch testing, to rule out other underlying conditions or identify any relevant allergies or irritants that may be contributing to the development of perioral dermatitis.

Recognizing the characteristic clinical features and applying the appropriate diagnostic criteria are essential for healthcare providers to accurately identify and manage this challenging skin condition.

Stages and Severity of Perioral Dermatitis

Perioral dermatitis can present with varying degrees of severity and may progress through different stages over time. Understanding the stages and the severity of the condition is crucial for healthcare providers to develop appropriate management strategies and monitor the patient's response to treatment.

Stages of Perioral Dermatitis

1. Early stage: In the early stage, the rash is typically confined to the skin immediately surrounding the mouth, with mild erythema, papules, and minimal scaling or dryness.
2. Intermediate stage: As the condition progresses, the rash may extend to the nasolabial folds, chin, and cheeks, with more pronounced erythema, scaling, and dryness.
3. Advanced stage: In the advanced stage, the rash may become more extensive, with the potential for the involvement of the nose and periocular area. The skin lesions may also become more inflamed and resistant to treatment.

Severity of Perioral Dermatitis

The severity of perioral dermatitis can be assessed based on the extent of the skin lesions, the intensity of the symptoms, and the impact on the patient's quality of life. Healthcare providers may use various assessment tools or grading systems to objectively evaluate the severity of the condition.

1. Mild perioral dermatitis: Characterized by a localized rash around the mouth, with minimal symptoms and a limited impact on the patient's quality of life.
2. Moderate perioral dermatitis: Moderate involvement of the skin, with more extensive lesions, increased symptoms, and a greater impact on the patient's quality of life.
3. Severe perioral dermatitis: Widespread and severe involvement of the skin, with significant inflammation, treatment resistance, and a substantial impact on the patient's quality of life.

It is important to note that the severity of perioral dermatitis can fluctuate over time, and individuals may experience periods of exacerbation and remission. Regular monitoring and assessment by healthcare providers are crucial for effective management and tailoring of treatment strategies to the individual's needs.

Management and Treatment Strategies

The management of perioral dermatitis typically involves a multifaceted approach, focusing on the identification and avoidance of potential triggers, the use of appropriate topical and systemic therapies, and the implementation of lifestyle modifications to promote skin healing and prevent recurrence.

Identification and Avoidance of Triggers

The primary goal in the management of perioral dermatitis is to identify and eliminate any potential triggers that may be contributing to the development or exacerbation of the skin condition.

1. Discontinuation of topical corticosteroids: If the patient has been using topical corticosteroids on the face, the healthcare provider will recommend the gradual discontinuation of these medications, as they can lead to the development or worsening of perioral dermatitis.
2. Avoidance of irritating cosmetic and personal care products: Patients should be advised to avoid products containing potential irritants, such as fragrances, preservatives, and occlusive ingredients, and instead use gentle, non-comedogenic formulations.
3. Identification of other potential triggers: Healthcare providers may work with patients to identify any other potential triggers, such as hormonal changes or environmental factors, that may be contributing to the condition and implement strategies to minimize exposure or manage the underlying factors.

Topical Treatments

The mainstay of treatment for perioral dermatitis involves the use of topical therapies to address the skin lesions and alleviate the associated symptoms.

1. Topical anti-inflammatory agents: Healthcare providers may prescribe low-potency topical corticosteroids, calcineurin inhibitors (e.g., tacrolimus, pimecrolimus), or azelaic acid to reduce inflammation and promote healing.
2. Topical antibiotics: In cases where there is a suspected secondary bacterial infection, topical antibiotic creams or gels containing ingredients like metronidazole or clindamycin may be used.
3. Topical sulfur-based products: Sulfur-containing preparations can help reduce the scaling and dryness associated with perioral dermatitis.

4. Gentle cleansers and moisturizers: The use of non-irritating, fragrance-free cleansers and moisturizers can help maintain the skin's barrier function and prevent further irritation.

Systemic Interventions

In more severe or recalcitrant cases of perioral dermatitis, healthcare providers may consider the use of systemic therapies to supplement the topical treatments.

1. Oral antibiotics: Oral antibiotics, such as tetracyclines or erythromycin, may be prescribed to address any underlying bacterial infections and modulate the inflammatory response.
2. Oral contraceptives or hormone therapy: In cases where hormonal factors are suspected to play a role, the healthcare provider may recommend the use of oral contraceptives or hormone therapy to help regulate the hormonal imbalances.
3. Oral retinoids: In some instances, oral retinoids, such as isotretinoin, may be considered for their anti-inflammatory and sebum-regulating properties, particularly in severe or treatment-resistant cases.

Lifestyle Modifications and Prevention

In addition to the medical treatments, healthcare providers should emphasize the importance of lifestyle modifications and preventive measures to help manage perioral dermatitis and reduce the risk of recurrence.

1. Gentle skin care: Recommending the use of mild, fragrance-free cleansers and moisturizers, and avoiding harsh scrubbing or exfoliation, can help maintain the skin's barrier function.
2. Sun protection: Encouraging the use of broad-spectrum sunscreen

can help prevent the exacerbation of perioral dermatitis and the development of post-inflammatory hyperpigmentation.

3. Stress management: Incorporating stress-reducing techniques, such as relaxation exercises, meditation, or counseling, may help mitigate the impact of stress on the condition.

4. Monitoring and follow-up: Regular follow-up with the healthcare provider, including monitoring for any potential triggers or recurrences, can help ensure timely intervention and management of the condition.

By implementing a comprehensive, multifaceted approach to the management of perioral dermatitis, healthcare providers can work collaboratively with patients to achieve better control over the condition, alleviate the associated symptoms, and prevent the recurrence of this challenging skin disorder.

Prognosis and Considerations

The prognosis for individuals with perioral dermatitis can vary depending on the severity of the condition, the patient's response to treatment, and the ability to identify and address any underlying triggers or contributing factors.

Prognosis

In general, the prognosis for perioral dermatitis is favorable, particularly when the condition is recognized and managed appropriately. With the discontinuation of topical corticosteroids, the use of appropriate topical and systemic therapies, and the implementation of lifestyle modifications, many patients can achieve good control over their skin condition and experience prolonged periods of remission.

However, in some cases, perioral dermatitis may be more persistent or recalcitrant to treatment, particularly when there are underlying factors, such as hormonal imbalances or chronic exposure to irritants, that are not adequately addressed. In these instances, the condition may require more intensive and prolonged management, with a higher risk of recurrence.

Considerations and Comorbidities

While perioral dermatitis is primarily a skin condition, healthcare providers should be mindful of the potential associations and comorbidities that may accompany this disorder.

1. Rosacea: There is a potential overlap between perioral dermatitis and rosacea, as both conditions can affect the facial skin and present with similar clinical features. In some cases, the two conditions may coexist or be difficult to differentiate.
2. Acne vulgaris: Perioral dermatitis can sometimes be mistaken for or coexist with acne, particularly in adolescents or young adults. The differences in the clinical presentation and the lack of comedones in perioral dermatitis can help distinguish the two conditions.
3. Atopic dermatitis: Individuals with a history of atopic dermatitis may be more prone to developing perioral dermatitis, particularly in the setting of topical corticosteroid use or exposure to other irritants.
4. Psychological impact: The visible nature of perioral dermatitis and the associated discomfort can have a significant impact on an individual's self-confidence, mental well-being, and quality of life. Addressing the psychological aspects of the condition is an important consideration in the overall management approach.

By recognizing the potential comorbidities and considering the unique aspects of each patient's presentation, healthcare providers can develop a personalized management plan that addresses the multifaceted nature of perioral dermatitis and optimizes the long-term outcomes for individuals living with this challenging skin condition.

Conclusion

Perioral dermatitis is a distinctive form of facial dermatitis that primarily affects the skin around the mouth, nose, and chin area. In this chapter, we have explored the underlying etiology and predisposing factors associated with the development of this condition, highlighting the role of topical corticosteroid use, cosmetic products, hormonal influences, and structural/anatomical characteristics of the perioral region.

We have delved into the characteristic clinical presentation of perioral dermatitis, including the distinctive perifollicular distribution of the skin lesions, the absence of comedones, and the sparing of the vermilion border. Understanding the diagnostic criteria and the various evaluation techniques employed by healthcare providers is crucial for ensuring accurate diagnosis and appropriate management.

The comprehensive management strategies for perioral dermatitis involve a combination of identifying and avoiding potential triggers, the use of topical and systemic therapies, and the implementation of lifestyle modifications to promote skin healing and prevent recurrence. Emphasizing the importance of gentle skin care and the management of any underlying factors further reinforces the holistic approach to the care of individuals with this challenging skin disorder.

By equipping healthcare providers with a thorough understanding of perioral dermatitis, this chapter aims to empower them to deliver effective and personalized care to patients, ultimately improving the quality of life for those affected by this perplexing and often distressing skin condition. The insights gained here will serve as a valuable foundation as we continue our exploration of the diverse forms of dermatitis.

CHAPTER 10

C hapter 10: Dermatitis in Special Populations

While the general principles of dermatitis management apply across various patient populations, there are certain unique considerations and adaptations required when addressing dermatitis in specific groups, such as infants and children, the elderly, and pregnant individuals. In this chapter, we will explore the distinct characteristics, risk factors, and management strategies for dermatitis in these special populations.

Dermatitis in Infants and Children

Infants and children are particularly susceptible to developing various forms of dermatitis, with atopic dermatitis (eczema) being one of the most common. Understanding the unique aspects of pediatric dermatitis is crucial for healthcare providers to ensure appropriate diagnosis, treatment, and prevention.

Epidemiology and Characteristics

Atopic dermatitis is the most prevalent form of dermatitis in infants and children, affecting up to 20% of this population worldwide. The condition typically manifests in early childhood, with the majority of cases presenting before the age of 5.

In infants and young children, the distribution and clinical presentation of atopic dermatitis may differ from that observed in adults. Lesions are often found on the cheeks, forehead, and extensor surfaces of the extremities, rather than the typical flexural areas affected in older children and adults.

Additionally, infants may present with a unique form of atopic dermatitis known as "cradle cap," characterized by a thick, yellow, greasy scale on the scalp. This early-onset variant of the condition often resolves by the first year of life but may be followed by the development of the more classic atopic dermatitis presentation.

Risk Factors and Comorbidities
Certain factors may increase the risk of developing dermatitis in infants and children, including:

1. Family history of atopic conditions: Children with a parental or sibling history of atopic dermatitis, asthma, or allergic rhinitis are at a higher risk of developing the condition.
2. Immune system immaturity: The infant and childhood immune system is still developing, making children more susceptible to inflammatory and allergic skin conditions.
3. Exposure to environmental triggers: Allergens, irritants, and changes in temperature or humidity can exacerbate dermatitis in young children.
4. Skin barrier dysfunction: Genetic and epigenetic factors can contribute to an impaired skin barrier, increasing the risk of developing dermatitis.
5. Viral and bacterial infections: Children are more prone to skin infections, which can worsen or complicate dermatitis.

It is important to note that young children with dermatitis may also be at an increased risk of developing other atopic conditions, such as food allergies, asthma, and allergic rhinitis, known as the "atopic march."

Management Considerations

The management of dermatitis in infants and children requires a tailored approach, considering the unique characteristics and needs of this population.

1. Gentle skin care: Recommending the use of mild, fragrance-free cleansers and moisturizers is crucial to maintain the delicate skin barrier of infants and children.
2. Topical therapies: Healthcare providers may prescribe low-potency topical corticosteroids or calcineurin inhibitors, with careful monitoring for potential side effects.
3. Dietary modifications: For infants and children with suspected food allergies, the healthcare provider may recommend dietary changes or the introduction of hypoallergenic formulas.
4. Infection prevention and management: Prompt treatment of any secondary skin infections, such as impetigo or molluscum contagiosum, is essential to prevent complications.
5. Psychological support: Addressing the emotional and social impact of dermatitis on the child and the family is important for overall well-being.
6. Parent/caregiver education: Empowering parents and caregivers with knowledge about dermatitis management, trigger avoidance, and skin care techniques is key for successful long-term outcomes.

Dermatitis in the Elderly

As individuals age, the skin undergoes various structural and functional changes that can predispose the elderly population to the development and exacerbation of dermatitis. Recognizing and addressing the unique aspects of geriatric dermatitis is crucial for healthcare providers to ensure appropriate management and improve the quality of life for older patients.

Epidemiology and Characteristics

Dermatitis, particularly seborrheic dermatitis and stasis dermatitis, is a common skin condition among the elderly population. The prevalence of seborrheic dermatitis has been reported to range from 3% to 5% in older adults, with an even higher incidence in those with underlying medical conditions or immunosuppression.

The clinical presentation of dermatitis in the elderly may differ from younger patients due to the age-related changes in the skin. Older individuals may exhibit more extensive, persistent, and treatment-resistant skin lesions, as well as an increased risk of complications, such as secondary infections and skin atrophy.

Risk Factors and Comorbidities

Several factors contribute to the increased susceptibility of the elderly population to the development and exacerbation of dermatitis, including:

1. Compromised skin barrier: Aging is associated with a decline in skin barrier function, leading to increased transepidermal water loss and susceptibility to irritants and allergens.
2. Impaired immune function: The aging immune system, known as immunosenescence, can contribute to the development and persistence of inflammatory skin conditions.
3. Underlying medical conditions: Chronic diseases common in the elderly, such as diabetes, cardiovascular disorders, and neurological conditions, can predispose individuals to the development of specific forms of dermatitis.
4. Polypharmacy and medication side effects: The use of multiple medications, particularly topical or systemic corticosteroids, can lead to the development or exacerbation of dermatitis.
5. Reduced mobility and self-care abilities: Physical limitations and cognitive decline in the elderly can make it challenging to maintain

proper skin hygiene and adhere to treatment regimens.

Management Considerations

The management of dermatitis in the elderly population requires a comprehensive and tailored approach, addressing the unique needs and challenges of this patient group.

1. Gentle skin care: Recommending the use of mild, fragrance-free cleansers and moisturizers, as well as the avoidance of irritants, is crucial to maintain skin health.
2. Topical therapies: Healthcare providers may need to adjust the potency and duration of topical corticosteroids or calcineurin inhibitors to avoid potential side effects, such as skin atrophy.
3. Systemic treatments: The use of oral or injectable medications, such as antihistamines or immunosuppressants, should be carefully evaluated and monitored in the elderly due to the increased risk of adverse effects and drug interactions.
4. Wound care and infection prevention: Prompt management of any skin infections or ulcerations is essential to prevent complications and promote healing.
5. Caregiver education and support: Involving and educating caregivers, family members, or nursing staff is crucial for ensuring proper skin care, medication adherence, and the implementation of preventive measures.
6. Multidisciplinary collaboration: A collaborative approach involving dermatologists, geriatric specialists, and other healthcare providers may be necessary to address the complex medical needs of elderly patients with dermatitis.

Dermatitis in Pregnancy

Pregnancy can significantly impact the development and progression of various skin conditions, including dermatitis. Understanding the unique aspects of dermatitis during pregnancy is important for healthcare providers to ensure the safe and effective management of this population.

Epidemiology and Characteristics

Pregnancy can influence the expression of certain forms of dermatitis, such as atopic dermatitis and seborrheic dermatitis. Atopic dermatitis, in particular, may improve, worsen, or remain unchanged during pregnancy, depending on the individual's hormonal and immunological responses.

Seborrheic dermatitis, on the other hand, is more commonly reported to worsen during pregnancy, with an increased prevalence and severity of the condition. This may be attributed to the hormonal changes and increased sebum production associated with pregnancy.

Risk Factors and Comorbidities

Pregnancy-related factors that can contribute to the development or exacerbation of dermatitis include:

1. Hormonal changes: The fluctuations in estrogen, progesterone, and other hormones during pregnancy can influence the skin's barrier function and immune responses.
2. Increased skin hydration and sebum production: Physiological changes in the skin, such as increased hydration and sebum secretion, can predispose pregnant women to the development of dermatitis.
3. Stress and emotional factors: The emotional and physical demands of pregnancy can trigger or worsen dermatitis through the modulation of the immune system and skin barrier.
4. Underlying medical conditions: Existing skin conditions, such as atopic dermatitis or seborrheic dermatitis, may be exacerbated during pregnancy.

Management Considerations

The management of dermatitis in pregnant women requires a delicate balance between ensuring the safety of the mother and the developing fetus, while also effectively addressing the skin condition.

1. Topical therapies: Healthcare providers may recommend the use of low-potency topical corticosteroids or calcineurin inhibitors, with careful monitoring and consideration of the potential impact on the fetus.
2. Systemic treatments: The use of systemic medications, such as oral antihistamines or immunosuppressants, should be thoroughly evaluated and discussed with the patient, as they may carry potential risks during pregnancy.
3. Skin care and lifestyle modifications: Emphasizing the importance of gentle skin care, hydration, and the avoidance of potential triggers can help manage dermatitis during pregnancy.
4. Emotional support and stress management: Addressing the emotional and psychological aspects of dermatitis, particularly during this life stage, can be beneficial for the overall well-being of the mother and the developing child.
5. Collaboration with obstetricians and other healthcare providers: A multidisciplinary approach, involving dermatologists, obstetricians, and other specialists, can help ensure the comprehensive and safe management of dermatitis in pregnant women.

It is important to note that the management of dermatitis during pregnancy may need to be adjusted based on the trimester, the severity of the condition, and the potential risks to the developing fetus. Regular monitoring and close communication between the patient and the healthcare team are essential to ensure the best possible outcomes for both the mother and the child.

Conclusion

Dermatitis can present unique challenges and considerations when encountered in special populations, such as infants and children, the elderly, and pregnant individuals. Understanding the distinct characteristics, risk factors, and management strategies for these patient groups is crucial for healthcare providers to deliver effective and personalized care.

In this chapter, we have explored the epidemiology, clinical features, and comorbidities associated with dermatitis in infants, children, the elderly, and pregnant women. We have highlighted the importance of tailored approaches to skin care, the use of appropriate topical and systemic therapies, and the need for caregiver education and multidisciplinary collaboration to address the unique needs and vulnerabilities of these special populations.

By equipping healthcare providers with the knowledge and insights presented in this chapter, we aim to empower them to navigate the complexities of dermatitis management in these specialized settings, ultimately improving the quality of life for patients and their families. The comprehensive understanding of dermatitis in special populations will serve as a valuable foundation as we continue our exploration of this diverse skin condition.

CHAPTER 11

Systemic Treatments for Dermatitis

While topical therapies play a crucial role in the management of dermatitis, there are instances where systemic interventions become necessary to achieve better control over the condition and improve the patient's overall quality of life. In this chapter, we will explore the various systemic treatment options for dermatitis, including oral antihistamines, immunosuppressants, and the emerging class of biologic therapies, as well as the key considerations and strategies for their effective and safe utilization.

Oral Antihistamines

Oral antihistamines are a class of systemic medications that can be used as an adjunct to the management of dermatitis, particularly in cases where the primary symptom is severe or debilitating pruritus (itching).

Mechanism of Action

Antihistamines exert their therapeutic effects by antagonizing the action of histamine, a key mediator of the inflammatory response and the primary driver of the itching sensation in dermatitis. By blocking the binding of histamine to its receptors, antihistamines can effectively alleviate the pruritus associated with various forms of dermatitis, including atopic dermatitis, contact dermatitis, and urticarial conditions.

Types of Oral Antihistamines

Oral antihistamines can be broadly classified into two generations:

1. First-generation antihistamines:
   - Examples: Diphenhydramine, hydroxyzine, and chlorpheniramine
   - Characterized by a higher potential for sedation and central nervous system (CNS) effects

2. Second-generation antihistamines:
   - Examples: Cetirizine, loratadine, fexofenadine, and desloratadine
   - Generally associated with a lower incidence of sedation and fewer CNS-related side effects

The selection of the appropriate oral antihistamine for patients with dermatitis should be based on the individual's tolerance, the desired effects (e.g., sedation vs. non-sedation), and the potential for drug interactions or adverse effects.

Clinical Applications in Dermatitis

Oral antihistamines can be beneficial in the management of dermatitis in the following scenarios:

1. Atopic dermatitis: Antihistamines can help alleviate the intense pruritus associated with this condition, particularly during acute flare-ups.
2. Contact dermatitis: They can provide symptomatic relief for the itching and hives that often accompany allergic contact dermatitis.
3. Urticarial conditions: Antihistamines are a mainstay in the management of chronic urticaria, which can be a comorbidity or a manifestation of certain forms of dermatitis.

In addition to their antipruritic effects, some antihistamines may also exhibit mild anti-inflammatory properties, potentially contributing to the overall management of dermatitis.

Dosing and Considerations

When prescribing oral antihistamines for the treatment of dermatitis, healthcare providers should consider the following:

1. Dosage and frequency: Antihistamines are typically dosed once or twice daily, with the specific dosage regimen depending on the individual medication and the patient's age and weight.
2. Sedative effects: First-generation antihistamines are more likely to cause drowsiness and impair cognitive function, which may be a concern for some patients. Second-generation antihistamines are generally preferred for their lower sedative profile.
3. Adverse effects: In addition to sedation, other potential side effects of oral antihistamines may include dry mouth, constipation, dizziness, and headaches.
4. Drug interactions: Certain antihistamines, particularly the first-generation agents, can interact with other medications, so healthcare providers should review the patient's medication history.
5. Caution in special populations: The use of oral antihistamines in children, the elderly, or individuals with underlying medical conditions (e.g., liver or kidney disease) may require dose adjustments or additional monitoring.

By carefully selecting the appropriate oral antihistamine and monitoring the patient's response and tolerability, healthcare providers can effectively incorporate these systemic medications into the comprehensive management of dermatitis.

Immunosuppressant and Immunomodulatory Agents

In cases of severe, refractory, or debilitating dermatitis, healthcare providers may consider the use of systemic immunosuppressant or immunomodulatory agents to help control the underlying inflammatory and autoimmune processes driving the condition.

Oral Corticosteroids

Oral corticosteroids, such as prednisone or prednisolone, are powerful anti-inflammatory and immunosuppressive agents that can be used to rapidly control the symptoms of severe or acute dermatitis flare-ups.

Mechanism of Action: Oral corticosteroids work by inhibiting the production and release of pro-inflammatory mediators, reducing the migration and activation of inflammatory cells, and modulating the immune system's response.

Indications and Use: Oral corticosteroids are typically reserved for the management of severe or debilitating dermatitis cases, such as:
  - Acute, widespread flare-ups of atopic dermatitis
  - Severe, recalcitrant cases of contact dermatitis
  - Erythrodermic or generalized forms of psoriatic dermatitis

Dosing and Duration: Oral corticosteroids are usually prescribed in a tapering regimen, starting with a higher dose and gradually reducing the dosage over time. The duration of treatment is often limited to the minimum necessary to achieve control of the dermatitis, typically ranging from a few days to a few weeks.

Adverse Effects and Considerations: Prolonged or inappropriate use of oral corticosteroids can lead to a wide range of adverse effects, including:
  - Metabolic disturbances (e.g., hyperglycemia, weight gain)
  - Cardiovascular complications (e.g., hypertension, fluid retention)
  - Musculoskeletal issues (e.g., osteoporosis, avascular necrosis)
  - Psychiatric and neurological effects (e.g., mood changes, insomnia)

- Increased susceptibility to infections

Healthcare providers must carefully weigh the potential benefits and risks of oral corticosteroid therapy, monitor the patient closely, and implement strategies to mitigate the adverse effects.

Steroid-Sparing Immunosuppressants

In cases where long-term control of dermatitis is required or when the use of oral corticosteroids is contraindicated or undesirable, healthcare providers may turn to alternative systemic immunosuppressant medications. These "steroid-sparing" agents can help manage the underlying inflammatory and autoimmune processes without the extensive adverse effects associated with chronic corticosteroid use.

Examples of systemic immunosuppressants used in the management of dermatitis include:

1. Methotrexate: A folic acid antagonist with anti-inflammatory and immunomodulatory properties, often used in the treatment of severe, recalcitrant cases of atopic dermatitis, psoriatic dermatitis, and other chronic, inflammatory skin conditions.
2. Azathioprine: A purine antimetabolite that suppresses the proliferation of T and B cells, commonly used in the management of severe, treatment-resistant atopic dermatitis or pemphigus.
3. Cyclosporine: A calcineurin inhibitor that disrupts T cell activation and cytokine production, effective in the management of severe atopic dermatitis and other inflammatory skin disorders.
4. Mycophenolate mofetil: An inhibitor of inosine monophosphate dehydrogenase, which can be used as a steroid-sparing agent in the treatment of various autoimmune and inflammatory skin conditions.

Mechanism of Action: These immunosuppressant medications work by targeting different aspects of the immune system, such as cell proliferation, cytokine production, and T cell activation, to modulate the underlying inflammatory and autoimmune processes driving dermatitis.

Indications and Use: Systemic immunosuppressants are typically reserved for patients with severe, recalcitrant, or debilitating forms of dermatitis that have not responded adequately to other treatment modalities, including topical therapies and oral antihistamines.

Dosing and Monitoring: The dosing and frequency of administration vary depending on the specific medication, the severity of the dermatitis, and the individual patient's response. Regular monitoring of laboratory parameters, such as blood counts, liver and kidney function, and drug levels, is crucial to ensure the safe use of these agents and to detect any potential adverse effects.

Adverse Effects and Considerations: Systemic immunosuppressants can be associated with a range of adverse effects, including:
- Increased risk of infections
- Gastrointestinal disturbances (e.g., nausea, diarrhea)
- Hepatotoxicity and nephrotoxicity
- Bone marrow suppression
- Increased risk of malignancies, particularly with long-term use

Healthcare providers must carefully balance the potential benefits and risks of these medications, closely monitor the patient, and implement appropriate strategies to mitigate the adverse effects.

Biologic Therapies

The field of dermatology has witnessed the emergence of a new class of systemic treatments known as biologic therapies. These novel agents, which are designed to target specific components of the immune system, have shown promising results in the management of various inflammatory and autoimmune skin conditions, including dermatitis.

Mechanism of Action

Biologic therapies are typically monoclonal antibodies or recombinant proteins that selectively target and modulate the activity of specific cytokines, receptors, or immune cells involved in the pathogenesis of dermatitis. By precisely intervening in the underlying immunological pathways, these agents can effectively reduce inflammation and improve the clinical manifestations of the skin condition.

Examples of Biologic Therapies in Dermatitis

Some of the biologic therapies currently approved or under investigation for the treatment of dermatitis include:

1. Dupilumab: A monoclonal antibody that targets the IL-4 and IL-13 cytokines, which play a central role in the pathogenesis of atopic dermatitis. Dupilumab is approved for the treatment of moderate to severe atopic dermatitis in adults and adolescents.
2. Tralokinumab: A monoclonal antibody that neutralizes the IL-13 cytokine, currently in clinical trials for the treatment of atopic dermatitis.
3. Lebrikizumab: A monoclonal antibody that targets the IL-13 cytokine, also being evaluated for the management of atopic dermatitis.
4. Nemolizumab: A monoclonal antibody that targets the IL-31 receptor, which is involved in the pathogenesis of pruritus associated with atopic dermatitis.
5. Tezepelumab: A monoclonal antibody that targets the thymic stromal lymphopoietin (TSLP) cytokine, currently in clinical trials for the treatment of atopic dermatitis.

Indications and Use

Biologic therapies are primarily indicated for the management of moderate to severe atopic dermatitis in patients who have not responded adequately to conventional treatments, such as topical therapies and systemic immunosuppressants.

These agents are typically administered by subcutaneous or intravenous injection, with the specific dosing and frequency of administration depending on the individual medication and the patient's response to treatment.

Advantages and Considerations

Biologic therapies offer several potential advantages in the management of dermatitis:

1. Targeted mechanism of action: By precisely targeting specific components of the immune system, biologic agents can provide more effective control of the underlying disease processes.
2. Improved safety profile: Compared to traditional systemic immunosuppressants, biologic therapies are generally associated with a lower risk of certain adverse effects, such as infection and organ toxicity.
3. Potential for long-term disease control: Biologic therapies may allow for sustained improvement and remission of the skin condition, reducing the need for continuous use of other systemic medications.

However, healthcare providers should also consider the following when prescribing biologic therapies for dermatitis:

1. Administration and monitoring: Biologic agents require specialized administration techniques and may necessitate close monitoring for potential adverse events, such as injection-site reactions or the development of antibodies.

2. Cost and access: Biologic therapies can be significantly more expensive than traditional systemic treatments, which may pose challenges in terms of access and affordability for some patients.
3. Long-term safety data: While the short-term safety profile of biologic therapies is generally favorable, the long-term effects, particularly in children and adolescents, are still being evaluated.

By carefully weighing the potential benefits and risks, healthcare providers can determine the appropriate role of biologic therapies in the comprehensive management of dermatitis, particularly in cases where conventional treatments have been ineffective or poorly tolerated.

Conclusion

Systemic treatments, including oral antihistamines, immunosuppressants, and biologic therapies, play a crucial role in the management of dermatitis, particularly in cases where topical therapies alone are insufficient or when the condition is severe, refractory, or debilitating.

In this chapter, we have explored the various systemic treatment options available for dermatitis, their mechanisms of action, indications, and key considerations for their safe and effective utilization. By understanding the appropriate application of these systemic interventions, healthcare providers can develop a comprehensive treatment plan that addresses the multifaceted aspects of dermatitis and improves the overall quality of life for patients.

As the field of dermatology continues to evolve, with the emergence of innovative biologic therapies, healthcare providers must remain vigilant in staying up-to-date with the latest advancements and evidence-based guidelines to ensure the delivery of optimal care for individuals living with this challenging skin condition.

By equipping healthcare providers with the knowledge and insights presented in this chapter, we aim to empower them to navigate the complexities of systemic dermatitis management, ultimately improving the outcomes and well-being of those affected by this chronic and often debilitating skin disorder.

CHAPTER 12

Complementary and Alternative Therapies for Dermatitis

While conventional medical treatments, including topical and systemic therapies, play a crucial role in the management of dermatitis, many patients also seek out complementary and alternative approaches to help alleviate their symptoms and improve their overall well-being. In this chapter, we will explore the various complementary and alternative therapies that have been explored or utilized in the context of dermatitis, examining their potential benefits, limitations, and the key considerations for their incorporation into a comprehensive treatment plan.

Dietary Modifications

The role of diet and nutrition in the management of dermatitis, particularly atopic dermatitis, has been an area of growing interest and research. Several dietary interventions and modifications have been investigated for their potential to influence the course of the skin condition.

Elimination Diets

One of the most common dietary approaches for atopic dermatitis is the implementation of elimination diets, which involve the removal of specific food allergens from the patient's diet. The rationale behind this approach is to identify and avoid trigger foods that may be contributing to the exacerbation of the skin condition.

Common food allergens that have been associated with atopic dermatitis include:
- Cow's milk
- Eggs
- Soy
- Wheat
- Peanuts
- Tree nuts

Healthcare providers may recommend that patients with suspected food allergies undergo allergy testing (e.g., skin prick tests, blood tests) to identify the specific triggers, which can then guide the implementation of an elimination diet. If a suspected food allergen is identified and removed from the diet, it may lead to an improvement in the patient's atopic dermatitis symptoms.

Anti-Inflammatory Diets

In addition to the elimination of specific food allergens, some patients with dermatitis may benefit from adopting an anti-inflammatory dietary approach. This type of diet aims to reduce the overall inflammatory burden by emphasizing the consumption of foods rich in anti-inflammatory nutrients, such as:

- Omega-3 fatty acids (e.g., fatty fish, flaxseeds, chia seeds)
- Antioxidants (e.g., fruits, vegetables, green tea)
- Probiotics (e.g., fermented foods, supplements)

The rationale behind an anti-inflammatory diet is to counteract the underlying inflammatory processes that contribute to the development and exacerbation of dermatitis. However, the evidence supporting the efficacy of this approach is still limited, and more research is needed to establish its benefits in the management of specific dermatitis subtypes.

Considerations and Limitations

While dietary modifications can be a valuable adjunct to the management of dermatitis, it is essential to consider the following:

1. Individualized approach: The effectiveness of dietary interventions can vary significantly among patients, so a personalized approach based on the individual's specific triggers and response is crucial.
2. Potential risks of elimination diets: Improperly implemented elimination diets can lead to nutritional deficiencies, particularly in children, and should be supervised by healthcare providers or registered dietitians.
3. Lack of robust evidence: While some studies have suggested potential benefits of dietary modifications, the overall evidence for their efficacy in dermatitis management is still limited and inconsistent.
4. Importance of conventional treatments: Dietary interventions should not replace conventional medical treatments, but rather be used as an adjunct to optimize the management of dermatitis.

Herbal and Botanical Remedies

The use of herbal and botanical remedies has a long-standing tradition in the management of various skin conditions, including dermatitis. While the scientific evidence supporting their efficacy is mixed, some of these natural therapies have shown promising results and may serve as complementary options for patients.

Topical Herbal Remedies

Several topical herbal and botanical preparations have been studied for their potential benefits in the management of dermatitis:

1. Colloidal oatmeal: Finely ground oats have been used as a soothing, anti-inflammatory, and emollient agent in the treatment of atopic dermatitis and other inflammatory skin conditions.
2. Chamomile: The anti-inflammatory and anti-bacterial properties of chamomile have been investigated for its potential use in the management of various forms of dermatitis.
3. Tea tree oil: This essential oil has been studied for its antimicrobial and anti-inflammatory effects, which may be beneficial in the treatment of certain types of dermatitis.
4. Aloe vera: The soothing and moisturizing properties of aloe vera have been explored for its potential use in atopic dermatitis and other inflammatory skin conditions.

Oral Botanical Supplements

In addition to topical applications, some patients with dermatitis may explore the use of oral botanical supplements as a complementary approach:

1. Omega-3 fatty acids: Supplements containing omega-3 fatty acids, such as fish oil or flaxseed oil, have been investigated for their anti-inflammatory effects in atopic dermatitis.
2. Quercetin: This flavonoid compound found in various fruits and vegetables has been studied for its potential anti-inflammatory and antioxidant properties in the context of dermatitis.
3. Turmeric (curcumin): The active compound in turmeric, curcumin, has been explored for its anti-inflammatory and antioxidant effects in the management of atopic dermatitis and other inflammatory skin conditions.
4. Probiotics: The use of probiotic supplements, which aim to modulate the gut microbiome, has been investigated for their potential benefits in atopic dermatitis and other inflammatory skin disorders.

Considerations and Limitations

When it comes to the use of herbal and botanical remedies for dermatitis, healthcare providers and patients should consider the following:

1. Lack of robust evidence: While some studies have suggested potential benefits of certain herbal and botanical therapies, the overall scientific evidence supporting their efficacy in the management of dermatitis is often limited or inconsistent.
2. Potential safety concerns: Some herbal and botanical products may interact with conventional medications or cause adverse reactions, particularly in individuals with underlying medical conditions or sensitivities.
3. Regulation and quality control: Herbal and botanical supplements are not subject to the same stringent regulatory oversight as conventional pharmaceutical products, which can make it challenging to ensure the quality, purity, and consistency of these preparations.
4. Importance of communication: It is crucial for patients to discuss the use of any herbal or botanical remedies with their healthcare providers, as these therapies should be used as a complement to, rather than a replacement for, conventional medical treatments.

Mind-Body Interventions

The impact of psychological and emotional factors on the development and progression of dermatitis has been increasingly recognized. As a result, various mind-body interventions have been explored as potential complementary therapies for individuals with this skin condition.

Stress Management Techniques

Chronic stress has been identified as a significant contributing factor in the exacerbation of dermatitis, particularly atopic dermatitis. Consequently, the incorporation of stress management techniques into the overall management of dermatitis has been a focus of research and clinical practice.

Examples of stress management techniques that may be beneficial for individuals with dermatitis include:
- Mindfulness-based practices (e.g., meditation, yoga, tai chi)
- Cognitive-behavioral therapy (CBT)
- Relaxation techniques (e.g., deep breathing, progressive muscle relaxation)
- Biofeedback

These mind-body interventions aim to help patients better manage their stress levels, which may in turn, contribute to the improvement of skin symptoms and overall well-being.

Psychotherapeutic Approaches

In addition to stress management, some healthcare providers may recommend psychotherapeutic approaches to address the emotional and psychological aspects of dermatitis, particularly in cases where the skin condition is significantly impacting the patient's quality of life.

Examples of psychotherapeutic interventions that may be beneficial for individuals with dermatitis include:
- Cognitive-behavioral therapy (CBT) to address negative thought patterns and coping strategies
- Psychodynamic therapy to explore the underlying emotional and psychological factors contributing to the skin condition
- Group therapy or support groups to provide a sense of community and shared experience among individuals with dermatitis

By addressing the emotional and psychological factors that may be associated with or exacerbating the dermatitis, these mind-body and psychotherapeutic interventions aim to provide a more comprehensive and holistic approach to the management of this skin condition.

Considerations and Limitations

When incorporating mind-body and psychotherapeutic interventions into the management of dermatitis, healthcare providers and patients should consider the following:

1. Individualized approach: The effectiveness of these interventions can vary significantly among patients, and a personalized approach tailored to the individual's specific needs and preferences is crucial.
2. Complementary role: Mind-body and psychotherapeutic approaches should be used as a complement to, rather than a replacement for, conventional medical treatments for dermatitis.
3. Accessibility and availability: Access to qualified practitioners trained in these specialized interventions may be limited in some healthcare settings, and the cost of these therapies may be a barrier for some patients.
4. Ongoing evaluation and monitoring: Healthcare providers should regularly assess the patient's progress and the impact of these complementary therapies on their overall dermatitis management and quality of life.

By recognizing the potential benefits of mind-body and psychotherapeutic interventions and incorporating them into a comprehensive treatment plan, healthcare providers can offer a more holistic approach to the management of dermatitis, addressing both the physical and psychological aspects of this chronic skin condition.

Prevention and Lifestyle Management

In addition to the various treatment modalities, the prevention and lifestyle management of dermatitis are crucial components in the overall approach to this skin condition. By empowering patients to adopt preventive measures and implement lifestyle modifications, healthcare providers can help reduce the risk of flare-ups, manage symptoms, and improve the long-term outcomes for individuals living with dermatitis.

Skin Care and Bathing Routines

Proper skin care and bathing practices are essential for maintaining the skin's barrier function and preventing the exacerbation of dermatitis. Healthcare providers may recommend the following guidelines:

1. Use of gentle, fragrance-free cleansers: Avoid harsh soaps, detergents, and other irritating products that can disrupt the skin's natural pH and barrier.
2. Lukewarm water temperature: Limit the use of hot water, which can strip the skin of its natural oils and lead to dryness.
3. Gentle drying: Pat the skin dry instead of rubbing, and avoid vigorous toweling.
4. Frequent application of emollients and moisturizers: The regular use of fragrance-free, hypoallergenic moisturizers can help restore the skin's barrier and prevent water loss.

Trigger Avoidance and Environmental Modifications

Identifying and minimizing exposure to potential triggers is a crucial aspect of dermatitis management. Healthcare providers may work with patients to:

1. Recognize and avoid specific allergens or irritants: This may include identifying and reducing exposure to environmental allergens, such as dust mites, pollen, or pet dander, as well as avoiding harsh chemicals, soaps, or other irritating substances.
2. Implement environmental modifications: This may involve changes to the home environment, such as using air purifiers, adjusting humidity levels, and selecting hypoallergenic bedding and clothing materials.

3. Manage stress and emotional factors: As stress can contribute to the exacerbation of dermatitis, healthcare providers may recommend stress-reducing techniques, such as mindfulness practices or counseling.

Dietary Considerations and Supplementation

As discussed in the previous section, dietary modifications and the use of certain supplements may play a role in the prevention and management of dermatitis. Healthcare providers may provide guidance on:

1. Elimination diets and identification of food triggers
2. Adoption of anti-inflammatory dietary approaches
3. Consideration of supplement use, such as omega-3 fatty acids or probiotics, to potentially support skin health

Ongoing Monitoring and Follow-up

Regular monitoring and follow-up with healthcare providers are crucial for the long-term management of dermatitis. This may involve:

1. Scheduled check-ins to assess the patient's skin condition, symptom control, and response to treatment
2. Adjustments to the treatment plan based on the patient's progress and changing needs
3. Screening for any associated conditions or complications that may develop over time

By empowering patients to take an active role in the prevention and lifestyle management of dermatitis, healthcare providers can help patients achieve better control over their skin condition, reduce the risk of flare-ups, and improve their overall quality of life.

Conclusion

Complementary and alternative therapies, including dietary modifications, herbal and botanical remedies, and mind-body interventions, can play a valuable role in the comprehensive management of dermatitis. While the scientific evidence supporting the efficacy of these approaches is still evolving, they may serve as important adjuncts to conventional medical treatments, providing patients with additional tools to address the multifaceted nature of this chronic skin condition.

In this chapter, we have explored the various complementary and alternative therapies that have been investigated or utilized in the context of dermatitis, examining their potential benefits, limitations, and the key considerations for their incorporation into a holistic treatment plan. We have also emphasized the crucial importance of prevention and lifestyle management strategies, including skin care, trigger avoidance, and dietary considerations, in the long-term management of dermatitis.

By equipping healthcare providers with the knowledge and insights presented in this chapter, we aim to empower them to engage in open and informed discussions with their patients about the role of complementary and alternative therapies, as well as the importance of preventive and lifestyle-based approaches. This comprehensive understanding will enable healthcare providers to develop personalized treatment strategies that address the diverse needs and preferences of individuals living with dermatitis, ultimately improving their overall health and quality of life.

As the field of dermatology continues to evolve, the integration of complementary and alternative therapies, alongside conventional medical treatments, holds the promise of a more holistic and patient-centered approach to the management of this challenging skin condition.

CHAPTER 13

Prevention and Lifestyle Management of Dermatitis

While the treatment of dermatitis often involves a combination of topical, systemic, and complementary therapies, the prevention and long-term management of this chronic skin condition rely heavily on the adoption of appropriate lifestyle strategies and preventive measures. In this chapter, we will explore the key aspects of dermatitis prevention and lifestyle management, equipping healthcare providers and patients with the knowledge and tools necessary to effectively manage this skin disorder and improve overall quality of life.

Skin Care and Bathing Routines

Maintaining proper skin care and bathing practices is a crucial component of dermatitis prevention and management. Healthcare providers should educate patients on the following guidelines:

1. Gentle cleansing:
   - Use fragrance-free, mild cleansers or emollient-based washes
   - Avoid harsh soaps, detergents, and exfoliating products that can disrupt
the skin's natural pH and barrier
   - Limit the frequency and duration of bathing or showering

2. Lukewarm water temperature:

- Bathe or shower in lukewarm water, as hot water can strip the skin of its natural oils and lead to dryness
- Limit the use of prolonged, hot soaking in baths

3. Gentle drying:
- Pat the skin dry gently instead of rubbing or vigorously toweling
- Avoid using rough or abrasive towels

4. Moisturization:
- Apply fragrance-free, hypoallergenic moisturizers immediately after bathing or showering to lock in hydration
- Use moisturizers liberally and consistently, even during periods of skin improvement

5. Targeted skin care for affected areas:
- For specific skin lesions or affected areas, healthcare providers may recommend the use of gentle, medicated cleansers or topical treatments as part of the daily skin care routine

By establishing and maintaining these gentle skin care and bathing practices, patients can help prevent further irritation, support the skin's natural barrier function, and reduce the risk of dermatitis flare-ups.

Trigger Avoidance and Environmental Modifications

Identifying and minimizing exposure to potential triggers is a crucial aspect of dermatitis management. Healthcare providers should work with patients to:

1. Recognize and avoid specific allergens or irritants:
- Environmental allergens: Dust mites, pollen, pet dander, or other airborne triggers
- Contact allergens: Chemicals, metals, fragrances, or other skin irritants

- Irritants: Harsh soaps, detergents, chemicals, wool, or synthetic fabrics

2. Implement environmental modifications:
- Use air purifiers or dehumidifiers to control indoor environmental triggers
- Choose hypoallergenic bedding, clothing, and other household materials
- Regularly clean and vacuum to reduce exposure to dust mites and other allergens

3. Manage stress and emotional factors:
- Recognize and address the role of stress, anxiety, and other psychological factors that may contribute to or exacerbate dermatitis
- Incorporate stress-reducing techniques, such as mindfulness, relaxation exercises, or counseling, into the patient's daily routine

By actively identifying and minimizing exposure to known triggers, patients can help prevent or reduce the frequency and severity of dermatitis flare-ups, ultimately improving their overall skin health and quality of life.

Dietary Modifications and Supplementation

The role of diet and nutrition in the management of dermatitis, particularly atopic dermatitis, has been an area of growing interest and research. Healthcare providers may recommend the following dietary strategies:

1. Elimination diets:
- Identify and eliminate specific food allergens, such as dairy, eggs, soy, or wheat, that may be contributing to the exacerbation of dermatitis
- Work with a healthcare provider or registered dietitian to ensure the elimination diet is safe and nutritionally adequate

2. Anti-inflammatory diets:
- Emphasize the consumption of foods rich in anti-inflammatory nutrients,

such as omega-3 fatty acids, antioxidants, and probiotics

- Limit the intake of pro-inflammatory foods, such as processed, high-fat, or high-sugar items

3. Dietary supplementation:

- Omega-3 fatty acids: Supplements containing fish oil or flaxseed oil may help reduce inflammation and improve skin barrier function

- Probiotics: Probiotic supplements may help modulate the gut microbiome and potentially influence the course of dermatitis

It is important to note that while dietary modifications and supplementation may be beneficial for some patients, the evidence supporting their efficacy in the management of dermatitis is still evolving. Healthcare providers should work closely with patients to implement these strategies in a safe and personalized manner, and not rely on them as a replacement for conventional medical treatments.

Protective Equipment and Clothing

Certain measures can be taken to protect the skin and prevent irritation in individuals with dermatitis:

1. Protective clothing:

- Choose breathable, natural fabrics (e.g., cotton, linen) that are less likely to cause irritation

- Avoid tight-fitting or synthetic clothing that can trap heat and moisture

- Use sun-protective clothing, such as long-sleeved shirts and pants, to prevent sun exposure

2. Gloves and protective barriers:

- Wear gloves when performing tasks that may expose the hands to irritants or allergens

- Use protective barriers, such as plastic gloves or sleeves, when handling household cleaners or other potentially irritating substances

3. Skin protection during activities:
   - Apply a thick layer of moisturizer or barrier ointment before engaging in activities that may cause skin irritation or friction
   - Consider using athletic tapes or bandages to protect affected areas during physical activity

By incorporating these protective measures into their daily routines, patients with dermatitis can help minimize the risk of flare-ups and further damage to the skin.

Stress Management and Psychological Support

The impact of psychological and emotional factors on the development and progression of dermatitis has been well-recognized. Healthcare providers should incorporate strategies for stress management and psychological support into the overall management plan.

Stress Management Techniques
   Chronic stress can exacerbate the symptoms of dermatitis and contribute to the development of flare-ups. Healthcare providers may recommend the following stress management techniques:

1. Mindfulness-based practices:
   - Meditation
   - Yoga
   - Tai chi

2. Relaxation exercises:
   - Deep breathing
   - Progressive muscle relaxation
   - Guided imagery

3. Cognitive-behavioral therapy (CBT):
  - Identify and modify negative thought patterns
  - Develop effective coping strategies

By incorporating these stress management techniques into their daily routine, patients can learn to better manage the psychological and emotional aspects of dermatitis, which may help improve their overall skin health and quality of life.

Psychological Support and Counseling

In addition to stress management, some patients may benefit from more formal psychological support or counseling. Healthcare providers should be prepared to:

1. Assess the patient's psychological well-being:
  - Evaluate the impact of dermatitis on the patient's mental health, self-esteem, and quality of life

2. Provide or refer for counseling or psychotherapy:
  - Cognitive-behavioral therapy (CBT) to address negative thought patterns and coping strategies
  - Psychodynamic therapy to explore underlying emotional and psychological factors
  - Support groups to provide a sense of community and shared experience

3. Collaborate with mental health professionals:
  - Work closely with mental health providers to ensure a comprehensive and coordinated approach to the patient's care

By addressing the psychological and emotional aspects of dermatitis, healthcare providers can help patients develop better coping mechanisms, improve their self-image and confidence, and ultimately enhance their overall well-being and ability to manage the skin condition.

Ongoing Monitoring and Prevention of Complications

Effective long-term management of dermatitis requires a proactive approach that includes regular monitoring, early intervention, and the prevention of potential complications.

Monitoring and Follow-up

Regular follow-up visits with healthcare providers are essential for the ongoing management of dermatitis. This may include:

1. Scheduled check-ins to assess the patient's skin condition, symptom control, and response to treatment
2. Adjustments to the treatment plan based on the patient's progress and changing needs
3. Screening for any associated conditions or complications that may develop over time

By maintaining regular contact with their healthcare providers, patients can ensure that any changes or exacerbations in their dermatitis are promptly addressed, and the treatment plan is continuously optimized to meet their evolving needs.

Prevention of Complications

Dermatitis, if left unmanaged or poorly controlled, can lead to the development of various complications. Healthcare providers should work with patients to implement strategies to prevent these complications, which may include:

1. Secondary skin infections:
- Prompt treatment of any bacterial, fungal, or viral skin infections that may arise

- Education on proper skin hygiene and wound care

2. Skin damage and scarring:
  - Encouraging the use of protective clothing and barriers to minimize skin trauma
  - Addressing any underlying factors that may contribute to skin damage, such as chronic scratching or excessive friction

3. Psychological and social impact:
  - Providing or referring patients to counseling or support services to address the emotional and social consequences of dermatitis
  - Empowering patients to advocate for themselves and navigate social or occupational challenges

4. Comorbidities and associated conditions:
  - Screening for and managing any underlying medical conditions that may be associated with or exacerbate dermatitis, such as atopic disorders, autoimmune diseases, or neurological conditions

By proactively addressing the potential complications of dermatitis, healthcare providers can help patients maintain better control over their skin condition, prevent further deterioration, and improve their overall quality of life.

Empowering Patients through Education and Shared Decision-Making

Effective prevention and long-term management of dermatitis require a collaborative approach between healthcare providers and patients. By empowering patients with knowledge and involving them in the decision-making process, healthcare providers can enhance the patient's engagement, adherence, and ultimately, the outcomes of dermatitis management.

Patient Education

Healthcare providers should prioritize patient education as a crucial component of dermatitis management. This may include:

1. Explaining the nature of the skin condition, its underlying causes, and the rationale for the recommended treatment approaches
2. Providing guidance on proper skin care, trigger avoidance, and lifestyle modifications to prevent flare-ups
3. Educating patients on the appropriate use and potential side effects of topical and systemic therapies
4. Offering resources and strategies for managing the psychological and emotional aspects of dermatitis

By empowering patients with a comprehensive understanding of their skin condition, healthcare providers can foster better adherence to the treatment plan and encourage active participation in the management of dermatitis.

Shared Decision-Making

Involving patients in the decision-making process is essential for the long-term success of dermatitis management. Healthcare providers should:

1. Discuss the available treatment options, their potential benefits, and any associated risks or drawbacks
2. Encourage patients to express their preferences, concerns, and goals for managing their dermatitis
3. Collaborate with patients to develop a personalized treatment plan that aligns with their individual needs, lifestyle, and values
4. Regularly review the treatment plan and make adjustments based on the patient's feedback and response

By engaging in shared decision-making, healthcare providers can build a stronger therapeutic alliance with patients, promote self-management, and ultimately, improve the overall outcomes of dermatitis treatment.

Conclusion

The prevention and lifestyle management of dermatitis are crucial components in the comprehensive approach to this chronic skin condition. By empowering patients to adopt appropriate skin care and bathing routines, minimize exposure to triggers, and implement dietary and stress management strategies, healthcare providers can help reduce the risk of flare-ups, manage symptoms, and improve the long-term outcomes for individuals living with dermatitis.

In this chapter, we have explored the key aspects of dermatitis prevention and lifestyle management, highlighting the importance of a holistic, patient-centered approach. We have emphasized the need for healthcare providers to educate patients, engage them in shared decision-making, and collaborate with them to develop personalized strategies that address the multifaceted nature of this skin condition.

By equipping healthcare providers with the knowledge and tools presented in this chapter, we aim to enable them to empower their patients to take an active role in the prevention and long-term management of dermatitis. This comprehensive understanding will help healthcare providers and patients work together to achieve better control over the condition, reduce the risk of complications, and ultimately, improve the overall quality of life for those affected by this chronic and often challenging skin disorder.

As the field of dermatology continues to evolve, the integration of prevention and lifestyle management strategies, alongside conventional medical treatments, holds the promise of a more holistic and patient-centered approach to the management of dermatitis.

CHAPTER 14

ystemic Treatments for Dermatitis

While topical therapies play a crucial role in the management of dermatitis, there are instances where systemic interventions become necessary to achieve better control over the condition and improve the patient's overall quality of life. In this chapter, we will explore the various systemic treatment options for dermatitis, including oral antihistamines, immunosuppressants, and the emerging class of biologic therapies, as well as the key considerations and strategies for their effective and safe utilization.

Oral Antihistamines

Oral antihistamines are a class of systemic medications that can be used as an adjunct to the management of dermatitis, particularly in cases where the primary symptom is severe or debilitating pruritus (itching).

Mechanism of Action

Antihistamines exert their therapeutic effects by antagonizing the action of histamine, a key mediator of the inflammatory response and the primary driver of the itching sensation in dermatitis. By blocking the binding of histamine to its receptors, antihistamines can effectively alleviate the pruritus associated with various forms of dermatitis, including atopic dermatitis, contact dermatitis, and urticarial conditions.

Types of Oral Antihistamines

Oral antihistamines can be broadly classified into two generations:

1. First-generation antihistamines:
   - Examples: Diphenhydramine, hydroxyzine, and chlorpheniramine
   - Characterized by a higher potential for sedation and central nervous system (CNS) effects

2. Second-generation antihistamines:
   - Examples: Cetirizine, loratadine, fexofenadine, and desloratadine
   - Generally associated with a lower incidence of sedation and fewer CNS-related side effects

The selection of the appropriate oral antihistamine for patients with dermatitis should be based on the individual's tolerance, the desired effects (e.g., sedation vs. non-sedation), and the potential for drug interactions or adverse effects.

Clinical Applications in Dermatitis

Oral antihistamines can be beneficial in the management of dermatitis in the following scenarios:

1. Atopic dermatitis: Antihistamines can help alleviate the intense pruritus associated with this condition, particularly during acute flare-ups.
2. Contact dermatitis: They can provide symptomatic relief for the itching and hives that often accompany allergic contact dermatitis.
3. Urticarial conditions: Antihistamines are a mainstay in the management of chronic urticaria, which can be a comorbidity or a manifestation of certain forms of dermatitis.

In addition to their antipruritic effects, some antihistamines may also exhibit mild anti-inflammatory properties, potentially contributing to the overall management of dermatitis.

Dosing and Considerations

When prescribing oral antihistamines for the treatment of dermatitis, healthcare providers should consider the following:

1. Dosage and frequency: Antihistamines are typically dosed once or twice daily, with the specific dosage regimen depending on the individual medication and the patient's age and weight.
2. Sedative effects: First-generation antihistamines are more likely to cause drowsiness and impair cognitive function, which may be a concern for some patients. Second-generation antihistamines are generally preferred for their lower sedative profile.
3. Adverse effects: In addition to sedation, other potential side effects of oral antihistamines may include dry mouth, constipation, dizziness, and headaches.
4. Drug interactions: Certain antihistamines, particularly the first-generation agents, can interact with other medications, so healthcare providers should review the patient's medication history.
5. Caution in special populations: The use of oral antihistamines in children, the elderly, or individuals with underlying medical conditions (e.g., liver or kidney disease) may require dose adjustments or additional monitoring.

By carefully selecting the appropriate oral antihistamine and monitoring the patient's response and tolerability, healthcare providers can effectively incorporate these systemic medications into the comprehensive management of dermatitis.

Immunosuppressant and Immunomodulatory Agents

In cases of severe, refractory, or debilitating dermatitis, healthcare providers may consider the use of systemic immunosuppressant or immunomodulatory agents to help control the underlying inflammatory and autoimmune processes driving the condition.

Oral Corticosteroids

Oral corticosteroids, such as prednisone or prednisolone, are powerful anti-inflammatory and immunosuppressive agents that can be used to rapidly control the symptoms of severe or acute dermatitis flare-ups.

Mechanism of Action: Oral corticosteroids work by inhibiting the production and release of pro-inflammatory mediators, reducing the migration and activation of inflammatory cells, and modulating the immune system's response.

Indications and Use: Oral corticosteroids are typically reserved for the management of severe or debilitating dermatitis cases, such as:
  - Acute, widespread flare-ups of atopic dermatitis
  - Severe, recalcitrant cases of contact dermatitis
  - Erythrodermic or generalized forms of psoriatic dermatitis

Dosing and Duration: Oral corticosteroids are usually prescribed in a tapering regimen, starting with a higher dose and gradually reducing the dosage over time. The duration of treatment is often limited to the minimum necessary to achieve control of the dermatitis, typically ranging from a few days to a few weeks.

Adverse Effects and Considerations: Prolonged or inappropriate use of oral corticosteroids can lead to a wide range of adverse effects, including:
  - Metabolic disturbances (e.g., hyperglycemia, weight gain)
  - Cardiovascular complications (e.g., hypertension, fluid retention)
  - Musculoskeletal issues (e.g., osteoporosis, avascular necrosis)
  - Psychiatric and neurological effects (e.g., mood changes, insomnia)

- Increased susceptibility to infections

Healthcare providers must carefully weigh the potential benefits and risks of oral corticosteroid therapy, monitor the patient closely, and implement strategies to mitigate the adverse effects.

Steroid-Sparing Immunosuppressants

In cases where long-term control of dermatitis is required or when the use of oral corticosteroids is contraindicated or undesirable, healthcare providers may turn to alternative systemic immunosuppressant medications. These "steroid-sparing" agents can help manage the underlying inflammatory and autoimmune processes without the extensive adverse effects associated with chronic corticosteroid use.

Examples of systemic immunosuppressants used in the management of dermatitis include:

1. Methotrexate: A folic acid antagonist with anti-inflammatory and immunomodulatory properties, often used in the treatment of severe, recalcitrant cases of atopic dermatitis, psoriatic dermatitis, and other chronic, inflammatory skin conditions.
2. Azathioprine: A purine antimetabolite that suppresses the proliferation of T and B cells, commonly used in the management of severe, treatment-resistant atopic dermatitis or pemphigus.
3. Cyclosporine: A calcineurin inhibitor that disrupts T cell activation and cytokine production, effective in the management of severe atopic dermatitis and other inflammatory skin disorders.
4. Mycophenolate mofetil: An inhibitor of inosine monophosphate dehydrogenase, which can be used as a steroid-sparing agent in the treatment of various autoimmune and inflammatory skin conditions.

Mechanism of Action: These immunosuppressant medications work by targeting different aspects of the immune system, such as cell proliferation, cytokine production, and T cell activation, to modulate the underlying inflammatory and autoimmune processes driving dermatitis.

Indications and Use: Systemic immunosuppressants are typically reserved for patients with severe, recalcitrant, or debilitating forms of dermatitis that have not responded adequately to other treatment modalities, including topical therapies and oral antihistamines.

Dosing and Monitoring: The dosing and frequency of administration vary depending on the specific medication, the severity of the dermatitis, and the individual patient's response. Regular monitoring of laboratory parameters, such as blood counts, liver and kidney function, and drug levels, is crucial to ensure the safe use of these agents and to detect any potential adverse effects.

Adverse Effects and Considerations: Systemic immunosuppressants can be associated with a range of adverse effects, including:
- Increased risk of infections
- Gastrointestinal disturbances (e.g., nausea, diarrhea)
- Hepatotoxicity and nephrotoxicity
- Bone marrow suppression
- Increased risk of malignancies, particularly with long-term use

Healthcare providers must carefully balance the potential benefits and risks of these medications, closely monitor the patient, and implement appropriate strategies to mitigate the adverse effects.

Biologic Therapies

The field of dermatology has witnessed the emergence of a new class of systemic treatments known as biologic therapies. These novel agents, which are designed to target specific components of the immune system, have shown promising results in the management of various inflammatory and autoimmune skin conditions, including dermatitis.

Mechanism of Action

Biologic therapies are typically monoclonal antibodies or recombinant proteins that selectively target and modulate the activity of specific cytokines, receptors, or immune cells involved in the pathogenesis of dermatitis. By precisely intervening in the underlying immunological pathways, these agents can effectively reduce inflammation and improve the clinical manifestations of the skin condition.

Examples of Biologic Therapies in Dermatitis

Some of the biologic therapies currently approved or under investigation for the treatment of dermatitis include:

1. Dupilumab: A monoclonal antibody that targets the IL-4 and IL-13 cytokines, which play a central role in the pathogenesis of atopic dermatitis. Dupilumab is approved for the treatment of moderate to severe atopic dermatitis in adults and adolescents.
2. Tralokinumab: A monoclonal antibody that neutralizes the IL-13 cytokine, currently in clinical trials for the treatment of atopic dermatitis.
3. Lebrikizumab: A monoclonal antibody that targets the IL-13 cytokine, also being evaluated for the management of atopic dermatitis.
4. Nemolizumab: A monoclonal antibody that targets the IL-31 receptor, which is involved in the pathogenesis of pruritus associated with atopic dermatitis.
5. Tezepelumab: A monoclonal antibody that targets the thymic stromal lymphopoietin (TSLP) cytokine, currently in clinical trials for the treatment of atopic dermatitis.

Indications and Use

Biologic therapies are primarily indicated for the management of moderate to severe atopic dermatitis in patients who have not responded adequately to conventional treatments, such as topical therapies and systemic immunosuppressants.

These agents are typically administered by subcutaneous or intravenous injection, with the specific dosing and frequency of administration depending on the individual medication and the patient's response to treatment.

Advantages and Considerations

Biologic therapies offer several potential advantages in the management of dermatitis:

1. Targeted mechanism of action: By precisely targeting specific components of the immune system, biologic agents can provide more effective control of the underlying disease processes.
2. Improved safety profile: Compared to traditional systemic immunosuppressants, biologic therapies are generally associated with a lower risk of certain adverse effects, such as infection and organ toxicity.
3. Potential for long-term disease control: Biologic therapies may allow for sustained improvement and remission of the skin condition, reducing the need for continuous use of other systemic medications.

However, healthcare providers should also consider the following when prescribing biologic therapies for dermatitis:

1. Administration and monitoring: Biologic agents require specialized administration techniques and may necessitate close monitoring for potential adverse events, such as injection-site reactions or the development of antibodies.

2. Cost and access: Biologic therapies can be significantly more expensive than traditional systemic treatments, which may pose challenges in terms of access and affordability for some patients.
3. Long-term safety data: While the short-term safety profile of biologic therapies is generally favorable, the long-term effects, particularly in children and adolescents, are still being evaluated.

By carefully weighing the potential benefits and risks, healthcare providers can determine the appropriate role of biologic therapies in the comprehensive management of dermatitis, particularly in cases where conventional treatments have been ineffective or poorly tolerated.

Conclusion

Systemic treatments, including oral antihistamines, immunosuppressants, and biologic therapies, play a crucial role in the management of dermatitis, particularly in cases where topical therapies alone are insufficient or when the condition is severe, refractory, or debilitating.

In this chapter, we have explored the various systemic treatment options available for dermatitis, their mechanisms of action, indications, and key considerations for their safe and effective utilization. By understanding the appropriate application of these systemic interventions, healthcare providers can develop a comprehensive treatment plan that addresses the multifaceted aspects of dermatitis and improves the overall quality of life for patients.

As the field of dermatology continues to evolve, with the emergence of innovative biologic therapies, healthcare providers must remain vigilant in staying up-to-date with the latest advancements and evidence-based guidelines to ensure the delivery of optimal care for individuals living with this challenging skin condition.

By equipping healthcare providers with the knowledge and insights presented in this chapter, we aim to empower them to navigate the complexities of systemic dermatitis management, ultimately improving the outcomes and well-being of those affected by this chronic and often debilitating skin disorder.

CONCLUSION

D ermatitis: A Multifaceted Challenge Requiring a Comprehensive Approach

Throughout this comprehensive guide, we have delved into the intricate and diverse world of dermatitis, exploring the various forms of this skin condition, their underlying causes, and the most effective management strategies. From the relentless itch of atopic dermatitis to the unsightly rashes of contact dermatitis, the journey has been one of uncovering the complexities that healthcare providers and patients alike must navigate when confronting this pervasive and often debilitating skin disorder.

As we reach the conclusion of this book, it is essential to emphasize the fundamental importance of a comprehensive approach to the management of dermatitis. While the specific manifestations and etiologies may vary, the common thread that unites these diverse skin conditions is the involvement of the skin's immune system, leading to a characteristic pattern of inflammation, redness, and discomfort. Recognizing and addressing the multifaceted nature of dermatitis is crucial for healthcare providers to deliver effective and personalized care, and for patients to achieve better control over their skin health and improve their overall quality of life.

The Power of Understanding: Empowering Healthcare Providers and Patients

The overarching goal of this book has been to empower both healthcare providers and patients with a comprehensive understanding of dermatitis, equipping them with the knowledge and tools necessary to navigate the complexities of this skin condition and ultimately improve outcomes.

For healthcare providers, the insights gained throughout the chapters have provided a solid foundation for accurately diagnosing, effectively managing, and closely monitoring individuals living with dermatitis. By understanding the intricate interplay between genetic, environmental, and immunological factors that contribute to the development and progression of these skin disorders, healthcare providers can tailor their approaches to the unique needs and characteristics of each patient.

Moreover, the detailed exploration of the various treatment modalities, including topical therapies, systemic interventions, and complementary approaches, has empowered healthcare providers to develop personalized treatment plans that address the multifaceted aspects of dermatitis. This comprehensive understanding enables them to make informed decisions, weigh the potential benefits and risks, and collaborate with patients to achieve the best possible outcomes.

For patients, this book has aimed to demystify the complexities of dermatitis, empowering them to take an active role in the management of their skin condition. By gaining a deeper understanding of the underlying causes, the various manifestations, and the available treatment options, patients can become more engaged in their own care, advocate for their needs, and work collaboratively with healthcare providers to develop effective strategies for long-term management and prevention.

Moreover, the emphasis on the psychological and emotional impact of dermatitis, as well as the importance of lifestyle modifications and preventive measures, has equipped patients with the knowledge and resources to address the holistic well-being considerations associated with this chronic skin disorder. This comprehensive approach empowers patients to adopt a more proactive and self-empowered stance in managing their dermatitis, ultimately improving their overall quality of life.

Navigating the Evolving Landscape of Dermatitis Management

As the field of dermatology continues to evolve, the management of dermatitis is poised to undergo significant advancements. The emergence of innovative treatment modalities, such as biologic therapies and targeted immunomodulatory agents, holds the promise of more effective and personalized care for individuals living with these skin conditions.

Additionally, the ongoing research into the underlying pathophysiology, genetic factors, and environmental triggers associated with dermatitis will undoubtedly lead to a deeper understanding of these skin disorders, enabling healthcare providers to refine their diagnostic and management approaches.

Furthermore, the growing emphasis on the integration of complementary and alternative therapies, as well as the recognition of the importance of preventive measures and lifestyle modifications, underscores the need for a holistic and patient-centered approach to the management of dermatitis. By embracing this multifaceted perspective, healthcare providers and patients can work together to optimize outcomes and improve the overall well-being of those affected by these challenging skin conditions.

The Role of Collaboration and Continuous Learning

Delivering effective and comprehensive care for individuals with dermatitis requires a collaborative effort among various healthcare professionals, including dermatologists, primary care providers, nurses, pharmacists, and allied health specialists. By fostering interdisciplinary collaboration and communication, healthcare teams can ensure a coordinated and well-rounded approach to the management of dermatitis, addressing the diverse needs and complexities that these patients may face.

Moreover, as the field of dermatology continues to evolve, it is essential for healthcare providers to maintain a commitment to continuous learning and professional development. Staying abreast of the latest research, guidelines, and emerging treatment modalities will empower them to provide the most up-to-date and evidence-based care for their patients with dermatitis.

Similarly, patients must be encouraged to actively engage with their healthcare providers, share their experiences, and participate in the decision-making process. This collaborative partnership between healthcare providers and patients is crucial for the successful management of dermatitis, as it enables the tailoring of treatment strategies to the unique needs and preferences of each individual.

The Path Forward: Improving Quality of Life and Reducing the Burden of Dermatitis

As we look to the future, the overarching goal in the management of dermatitis must be to improve the quality of life for those affected by these skin conditions and to reduce the significant burden they place on individuals, families, and the healthcare system as a whole.

By equipping healthcare providers and patients with the comprehensive knowledge and strategies outlined in this book, we aim to empower them to navigate the complexities of dermatitis with confidence, empathy, and a commitment to holistic care. Through accurate diagnosis, personalized treatment approaches, and the integration of preventive measures and lifestyle modifications, we can strive to achieve better control over these skin disorders, alleviate the associated symptoms and discomfort, and ultimately enhance the overall well-being of those living with dermatitis.

Moreover, the continued advancement in research, the development of innovative therapies, and the fostering of collaborative healthcare teams will be instrumental in driving progress in the management of dermatitis. As we navigate this evolving landscape, it is essential that we remain vigilant, adaptable, and dedicated to providing the highest quality of care to our patients.

Conclusion

Dermatitis, with its diverse manifestations and complex etiologies, remains a significant challenge in the field of dermatology. However, through the comprehensive understanding and the multifaceted management strategies presented in this book, we are confident that healthcare providers and patients can work together to overcome the hurdles and improve the lives of those affected by these skin conditions.

By empowering healthcare providers with the knowledge and tools necessary to deliver effective and personalized care, and by equipping patients with the understanding and resources to take an active role in the management of their dermatitis, we hope to foster a collaborative and patient-centered approach that ultimately leads to better outcomes and enhanced quality of life.

As we look to the future, the continued commitment to research, innovation, and interdisciplinary collaboration will be crucial in driving progress in the field of dermatitis management. By embracing this comprehensive and evolving approach, we can strive to alleviate the burden of dermatitis and provide hope and support to the millions of individuals who struggle with these challenging skin conditions.